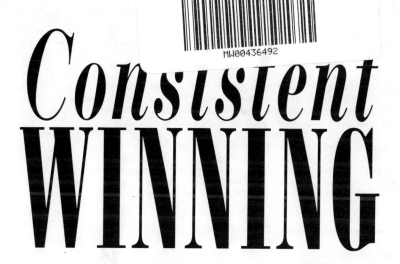

Consistent WINNING

A Remarkable New Training System That Lets You Peak on Demand

By Ronald D. Sandler, D.P.M.
and Dennis D. Lobstein, Ph.D.

Rodale Press, Emmaus, Pennsylvania

Dedication

With loving thanks to Sylvia Sandler, Herbert Sandler, Miriam Lobstein, and Otto Lobstein, whose help and devotion made this book possible.

Printed in the United States of America on acid-free ∞ paper

Editor: Sara J. Henry
Book designer: Lisa Farkas
Cover designer: Stan Green
Illustrator: Ruttle, Shaw & Wetherill, Inc.
Copy Editor: Ellen Pahl
Indexer: Ed Yeager

Photo credits: Ronald D. Sandler, pages 18–19 and 29 (starfish, shefflera, daisy, shell, nautilus)
National Oceanic and Atmospheric Administration, DOC/NESDIS/SCSC, page 26 (hurricane)
California Association for Research in Astronomy/CARA, page 28 (galaxy)
Heritage House '76, Inc., page 29 (fetus)

If you have any questions or comments concerning this book, please write:
Rodale Press
Book Readers' Service
33 East Minor Street
Emmaus, PA 18098

Library of Congress Cataloging-in-Publication Data

Sandler, Ronald D.
    Consistent winning : a remarkable new training system that lets
you peak on demand / by Ronald D. Sandler and Dennis D. Lobstein.
        p.   cm.
    Includes bibliographical references (p.   ) and index.
    ISBN 0–87596–134–7 paperback
    1. Physical education and training—United States.   2. Physical
education and training—United States—Psychological aspects.
    3. Running—United States—Training.   I. Lobstein, Dennis D.
II. Title.
GV203.S26   92–20011
613.7'172—dc20   CIP

Distributed in the book trade by St. Martin's Press

2 4 6 8 10 9 7 5 3 1   paperback

CONTENTS

ACKNOWLEDGMENTS

We extend our appreciation to the following athletes and friends who helped make possible or who assisted with *Consistent Winning:* Edmund Coccagna, Robert Prechter, Lyn Brooks, Scott Morson, Phil Kiner, John Dietrich, Nick Bassett, Jim Woodard, Nate Breen, Rich Ryan, Kit Carpenter, Ray Hosler, Bill Morris, Dr. Fred Waldman, Dr. Marc Spector, Dr. Jonathan Hyman, Dawn Heinsbergen, Irene Levitt, Lucy Jelinek, Don Stambler, Christy Anthony, Robert Sandler, Dr. Dale Rosenblum, Dee Britton, Claudia Suzanne Stein, Carol Amato, Lester Gottlieb, Kent Runge, and Sara Henry.

And special thanks to Herbert Sandler, Jill Lobstein, and Dr. A. H. Ismail.

INTRODUCTION

Why is it that sometimes when you train hard and feel fine, you have a good day—but other times when you train just as hard and feel just as fine, you have a bad day? And at other times, you do so well you wonder where it came from?

If you've ever trained for any event or competition, chances are you've noticed these wide variations in your day-to-day performance and energy levels. Why does this happen? Where does this surprising energy—or unexpected lethargy—come from? Why is it unpredictable? How can it be controlled?

Just about every athlete has wondered about this, and *Consistent Winning* gives you the answers. It presents an innovative new training technique that can be used for any activity. Any recreational or professional athlete, dancer, singer, or musician, or anyone who practices anything regularly and desires to improve, can use it. Performing artists, fine artists, programmers, and anyone involved in mental activities can benefit, as can anyone who is interested in maximum performance.

Consistent Winning explains, in understandable language, why peak performances occur and how to control them. If you use the Consistent Winning technique, you can obtain maximum performances exactly when you want them, while avoiding injury, illness, and burnout along the way.

What's unique about this technique is that it creates training cycles based on natural physiological cycles under your control—while changing nothing in your actual training. Using Consistent Winning is easy. All you have to do is follow the schedules of when to rest and when to train.

Consistent Winning helps anyone, whether beginner or elite athlete, or artist or musician, to stay healthy and to achieve peak performance when planned. And on event day, when you're pushing yourself to the limit, you may find that the limit is greater than you ever hoped for.

CHAPTER ONE

CAPTURING
THE ELUSIVE PEAK

It was the third day of the Ultraman Triathlon in Hawaii, 1984. The contestants had completed 6 miles of swimming and 90 miles of bicycling on the first day of the event, followed by 160 miles of bicycling the next day. Lyn Brooks, veteran triathlete, was feeling good the morning of the third day, as she prepared for the final leg of the Ultraman, the 53-mile double marathon run.

Completing the grueling run in the heat and humidity of Hawaii was not the only challenge facing Brooks. She was beginning the third day of competition in last place. Nevertheless, that day she ran 53 miles virtually nonstop and passed every female competitor to win the women's division.

Brooks's peak performance on the third day of the event was no accident: She had carefully planned to peak that day. It was, in fact, the fourth consecutive time she had achieved peak performance for a major event exactly on time, according to a prescheduled plan. Lyn Brooks had captured the elusive peak.

Her confidence in hitting a peak on the crucial day came not just from positive thinking or visualization, or from the knowledge that she had put in plenty of long, hard training hours. Brooks knew she would have a maximum performance day when planned

1

because she had carefully modified her training schedule according to the Consistent Winning technique.

A Program Anyone Can Use

Consistent Winning is a program of specific cycles of resting and training, developed after studying athletes and their patterns of training, injuries, time off, and peak performances. The cycles are based on a mathematical sequence known as Fibonacci numbers, which occur frequently in nature. (Fibonacci numbers are explained fully in chapter 3.)

All athletes—whether recreational or competitive—can benefit from Consistent Winning. It helps avoid injury, illness, and burnout by reducing physiological as well as psychological stress. With Consistent Winning, you can not only predict but actually schedule your peak performance days consistently and reliably.

Consistent Winning doesn't change or replace any established, viable program of workouts. It merely structures your given training schedule so you can schedule peak performances to occur on specific days. It's easy, safe, and convenient.

It's All in the Timing

Every coach, trainer, and athletic expert has an opinion on how many pounds, miles, sets, strokes, and practice games are necessary to prepare for peak performance. And there are literally thousands of athletes who faithfully run, swim, bike, lift, stretch, and struggle to achieve that peak, only to have their hoped-for burst of energy come a day late or two days early—any time except the right time. It's immensely frustrating when, after long, hard months of effort, they find themselves in the middle of a competition and they "just don't have it."

When this happens, athletes or coaches tend to blame themselves for overlooking something or not training enough even though they have developed healthy, effective training programs.

If you don't experience peak performances when you want them, that doesn't necessarily mean there's something wrong with the way you train.

What may be wrong is not *how* you're training but *when* you're training—and when you're resting.

Creating Your Peak

Consistent Winning allows you to schedule your peak performances by using cycles of training unlike any you've ever purposely used before—although you may well have accidentally happened upon them during your athletic endeavors. There are three basic cycles, all composed of a resting period and a training period, and each cycle is named for the *length of the training period*: 3-Day Cycle, 3-Week Cycle, and 3-Month Cycle.

Each cycle is designed to bring you to peak performance on

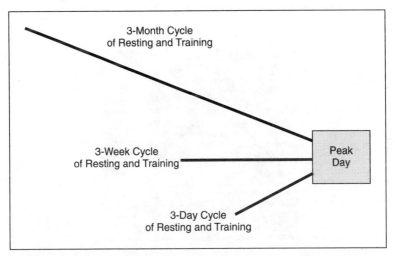

Consistent Winning Cycles: *Depending on how much time you have before your event, you can pick the 3-Day Cycle, 3-Week Cycle, or 3-Month Cycle. All lead to a peak performance on the final day of the cycle.*

PEAKS AND VALLEYS IN AN IRONMAN

Dave Scott, veteran triathlete and six-time winner of the Ironman Triathlon, may have unknowingly used the Consistent Winning technique—which involves specifically timed rest and workout cycles—en route to his 1986 and 1987 Ironman victories.

Because of many speaking engagements and other commitments before the 1986 event, Scott found himself forced to take off many periods of three to five days. "The more time I missed, the better I did," he said. "After about five days off I felt lethargic and stiff, but then I felt better in training than before."

At the 1986 Ironman, Scott turned in a course record. The next year his busy schedule continued to interfere with his training. "I missed many sets of days before the 1987 Ironman—more than in 1986," he said.

His winning time in 1987 was 5 minutes off his course record from the year before, but difficult weather conditions made it a tougher event. It was, Scott said, his best race so far. His "accidental" resting periods had paid off.

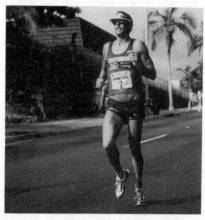

Man of Iron: *Dave Scott, here en route to his record-setting 1986 Ironman win, is a prime example of the benefits of resting periods.*

CHAPTER TWO

DISCOVERING CYCLES IN SPORTS PERFORMANCE

Consistent Winning is a unique training technique with training and resting periods in specific cycles that correlate to your own natural patterns. Here's how the concept occurred to author Ronald Sandler, D.P.M., and how he developed and tested Consistent Winning.

As a podiatrist, I work with many athletes, especially runners, who tend to overtrain and get hurt. During the late 1970s and early 1980s, I became aware that most of my athletic patients had certain buildup and breakdown cycles with their injuries—peaks and valleys, similar to the peaks and valleys in training and performance. In a valley, they would have an injury. During a peak, they were fine. It occurred to me that there might be a definable pattern to these peaks and valleys.

Injuries Don't Occur Randomly

Steve, one of my patients, was an avid runner. One day he suddenly and arbitrarily increased his daily 5-mile run to 8 miles. Three weeks after the new regimen, he was limping; a few days later he was in my office. It had taken exactly three weeks of his new program for his body to break down.

As time went by, I noticed similar patterns of illness and injury in many other athletes I treated. It was obvious that there were definite cycles to the injuries and the peaks, and that these cycles involved groups of weeks and days in threes and fives. It was also clear that a specific proportion of time was involved in each cycle, and that the cycles were in proportion to each other.

In Steve and in other patients, I could see that their cycles of buildup and breakdown and high and low performances seemed to conform to a certain pattern, and kept occurring in cycles of three and five weeks.

Defining the Patterns

When studying investments a few years earlier, I had learned about the Elliott Wave Principle, a pattern of natural advances and regressions used to help predict movements in the stock market. The Elliott Wave is derived from patterns in nature—including human nature—and Fibonacci numbers. From studying the Elliott Wave, I learned about Fibonacci numbers and the distinctive patterns in nature that are based on those numbers and their proportion to each other. (More about this in chapters 3 and 4.) I began to suspect that there was a correlation between human physical effort and these concepts as well.

More evidence of specific patterns came from one of my patients, Scott Morson, a triathlete from Cheyenne, Wyoming, who at the time was training for his third Ironman Triathlon. The Ironman Triathlon in Hawaii consists of a 2.4-mile ocean swim, a 112-mile bike race, and a 26.2-mile marathon run. Anyone who plans to compete in this event generally trains frequently, at least once and often twice a day.

One morning, Morson mentioned that he had done exceptionally well in a recent Boston Marathon and said, "I wish I could peak like that all the time." I said, "Do me a favor. Keep a record of how you feel and how you perform in your daily

WHAT ARE FIBONACCI NUMBERS?

Fibonacci numbers, first described by Leonardo Fibonacci in the thirteenth century, are a series of numbers that occur frequently in nature—in the number of petals on a flower, the ridges on a shell, and the legs on a spider, for example. Spiral forms based on these numbers can be seen in shells, hurricanes, the swirl of water going down a drain, and the curl of an ocean wave. Specific proportions based on these numbers are also used frequently in art and architecture, ranging from the Parthenon to Michaelangelo's _David._

This series of numbers was once thought to be nothing more than an interesting quirk of nature, but scientists in many areas are now beginning to appreciate the significance of this pervasive natural sequence. In addition to artists, musicians, and poets, scientists such as physiologists, biochemists, botanists, and computer scientists have acknowledged and made use of this naturally occurring phenomenon.

Curious? In chapter 3 you'll find further explanation of these numbers, their forms, and how they are used.

training." I didn't, however, explain why I wanted him to keep the records. He agreed.

Eight months later Morson gave me his daily records, and when I examined them I found specific and precise cycles. After three weeks of training, he hit a peak, then caught a cold. After another five weeks of training he peaked and then was injured. Exactly three more weeks of training ended with a peak performance. Athletic performance evidently did conform to a mathematical structure, and was predictable—at least for Scott Morson. Would the theory hold up with other athletes as well?

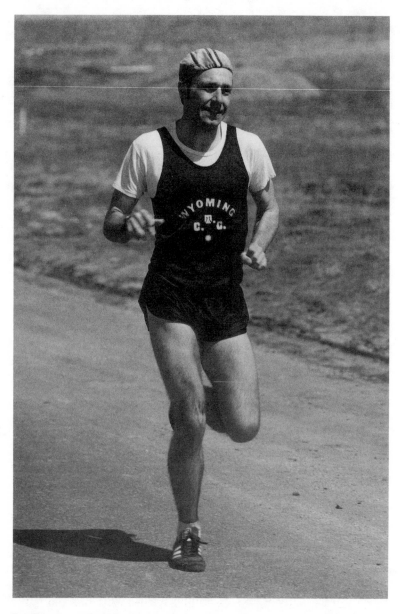

Performance Cycles: Scott Morson, a triathlete from Wyoming, was one of the first users of Consistent Winning.

The Theory Tests True

I made contact with 30 athletes I knew who trained daily, and asked them to keep records. I had them rate their days subjectively on a scale of 1 to 5, with "5" being an exceptional performance, "3" an average day, and "1" a day when they could barely get through the workout. I also asked them to take their resting pulse when they first awakened in the morning, both to see how well their bodies were recovering when close to a peak and to camouflage my motives. This was a blind test—none of the athletes knew what I was looking for or the reason for my observations.

After six months, ten of the original group supplied me with detailed records, and all showed the same pattern demonstrated in Morson's records—injuries and strong performances occurring in cycles of three and five weeks. I traveled to the next Ironman to observe Morson's performance and happened to meet Lyn Brooks, from Baltimore. Brooks was an excellent athlete who had placed third in the 1981 and February 1982 Ironman competitions and first in other international triathlons. She trained daily and kept meticulous records.

Without telling her why, I asked her to rate her days subjectively and send the records to me monthly. She agreed, and after four months I could see a clearly evident pattern in her monthly records.

I flew to Baltimore to meet with Brooks and explained the Consistent Winning technique. I pulled out her own forms to show how the records she had kept reflected the same patterns. She had never taken a rest, but every three weeks almost to the day—in fact usually exactly 21 days—she would have a top performance. *Every three weeks.* It convinced her to give the system a try. In the next 12 months she used the 3-Week Cycle—and peaked on her planned days four out of five times, an 80 percent success rate. Her Consistent Winning–aided finishes included the win at the Ultraman, a second in the Ultimate Triathlon in Sacramento, and, despite an accident during the race, a fifth in the Ironman in Nice, France.

Lyn Brooks—January 1983

S	M	T	
2 R—7 mi. (2 flats; B—8 mi. had to W—1 hr. stop) SB—1 hr. P=46 DR=4	**3** R—14 mi. SB—1 hr. S—1 mi. P=48 DR=4	**4** R—20 mi. W—1 hr. (best 20 since being sick) P=46 DR=4	**5** R—7 mi. SB—11/2 hr. S—1 mi. P=46 DR=4
9 R—7 mi. W—1 hr. SB—1/2 hr. S—1 mi. P=46 DR=4	**10** R—14 mi. W—1 hr. SB—1 hr. S—1 mi. P=44 DR=3	**11** R—20 mi. SB—1 hr. S—1 mi. P=46 DR=3	**12** R—7 mi. B—22 mi. W—1 hr. P=45 DR=3
16 R—7 mi. SB—11/2 hr. S—1 mi. P=48 DR=4	**17** (really up R—14 mi. day; not W—1 hr. necessarily SB—1 hr. great speed S—1 mi. but felt good) P=48 DR=5	**18** (slow; R—20 mi. very cold) SB—1/2 hr. S—1 mi. sprint P=50 DR=3	**19** R—7 mi. W—1 hr. SB—11/2 hr. S—1 mi. P=48 DR=31/2
23 R—10 mi. (10 mi. SB—1 hr. race; S—1/2 mi hilly; 69:55; felt good) P=46 DR=4	**24** R—14 mi. W—1 hr. SB—1 hr. S—1 mi. P=50 DR=4	**25** R—20 mi. SB—1/2 hr. S—1 mi. sprint P=50 DR=4	**26** R—7 mi. SB—11/2 hr. W—1 hr. S—1 mi. P=54 DR=3

**(R=run, B=bike, W=weights, SB=stationary bike, S=swim,
P=pulse, DR=day rating)**

Recorded Patterns: *Detailed record sheets, such as this one from Lyn
Brooks, were used to help develop the Consistent Winning technique.
Athletes recorded their workouts and rated each day on a scale of 1 to
5, with "5" being a great day and "3" an average day.*

Trying It Myself

I noted that the same sequences of performance were to be
found in my own daily records of running and bicycling, but I
decided to give the technique a more difficult test. For a long
time I had wanted to do a century, a 100-mile bicycle ride, but I
had never ridden more than 30 miles at a time. Using the Consis-

tent Winning technique, I trained for three months, doing three days a week on a bicycle and three days a week lifting weights. My longest rides were 30 miles once a week, except for a 40-mile ride and a 50-miler, done approximately three weeks and then two weeks before the event.

Finally, the day of the century arrived.

At 80 miles, I was averaging a faster speed than I ever accomplished on any of my 30-mile rides—and I felt great. At 85 miles, I was laughing: I didn't know where my energy was coming from!

Those very words came to my mind as I pedaled; it wasn't until later that I realized they were virtually the exact ones Lyn Brooks had used earlier when we discussed her peak performances: "I don't know where it came from." At 90 miles, I was thinking to myself, "Where is this coming from? Where am I getting this?" It was very exciting—the system was working. The peak was planned for, and there it was—what a feeling of power and control!

I have used Consistent Winning ever since for events such as bicycle centuries and have consistently avoided injury, illness, and burnout. The results have been great rides and consistent progress. Several times it had seemed that I was attempting an event beyond my abilities, but the technique has always come through.

CHAPTER THREE

UNLOCKING NATURAL PATTERNS

The precise timing of the resting and training cycles that make up Consistent Winning is based on Fibonacci numbers, a series of numbers that describes many naturally recurring phenomena. These numbers are an infinite sequence that pop up in both nature and art with amazing frequency; they form patterns that were first described 4,500 years ago. The series of numbers itself was first discovered and described by Leonardo Fibonacci some 800 years ago.

The Man behind the Magic

Fibonacci helped change the face of Western mathematics and civilization by bringing the simplicity of Arabic numbers to a world familiar only with Roman numbers. Born in Pisa toward the end of the twelfth century, he grew up in the North African city of Bugia, where his father was stationed as a customs official. There the Muslims along the Barbary Coast exposed Fibonacci to the concept of Arabic numbers. He was mesmerized by the ease of writing "98" instead of "XCVIII." It made all numerical tasks easier: drawing up a list, telling time, or performing any calculation, simple or complex.

Even after Fibonacci returned to Pisa as a young, inquisitive student, he was captivated by mathematical speculation, often becoming so involved in thoughts and equations that he would absentmindedly scrawl numbers onto whatever wall was closest when inspiration hit. This so exasperated his neighbors that they gave him a nickname: "Bigollone"—the Blockhead.

But in 1202, at age 27, Fibonacci published _Liber Abaci (The Book of the Abacus)_. It became the primary introductory source of Arabic numbers to the European world and made Fibonacci's fortune. His countrymen, now impressed with his accomplishments, awarded him the rare honor of living in one of the three Pisa towers.

As profound a contribution as Arabic numbers were, Fibonacci gave the Western world far more. In one section of his book, he described a simple mathematical puzzle whose solution resulted in a particular series of numbers we now call Fibonacci numbers (see "Fibonacci Rabbits" on page 17). This sequence, dubbed

---

MATHEMATICALLY DISINCLINED?

If at this point your mind's whirling with numbers, don't despair. You don't _have_ to understand Fibonacci numbers or the golden ratio to use the Consistent Winning technique. You don't even have to understand the Elliott Wave Principle (explained in chapter 4), which is how we relate Fibonacci numbers to sports performance.

Understanding these two concepts, however, _will_ help you understand why the resting and training cycles of Consistent Winning are so specific and why they work.

But if numbers make your head ache and graphs have you pulling out your hair—and you're willing to take our word that the cycles _do_ work without understanding why—you can skip directly to chapter 5, where the explanation of the Consistent Winning resting and training cycles begins.

the "Fibonacci summation sequence" by French mathematician Edouard Lucas in the nineteenth century, has since dazzled the imagination of generations upon generations of scientists, as more and more examples of it are found throughout nature and the universe. The depth and detail of Fibonacci's discovery is greater than can be thoroughly explored in this book, but the general idea is fascinating and useful.

Fibonacci Numbers: They're Everywhere!

Poring over the calculations that Fibonacci used to solve his rabbit puzzle isn't necessary (see "Fibonacci Rabbits" on the opposite page). What's exciting is the result, the series of numbers we now call Fibonacci numbers: 1; 1; 2; 3; 5; 8; 13; 21; 34; 55; 89; 144; 233; 377; 610; 987; 1,597; 2,584; 4,181; 6,765; 10,946; 17,711; 28,657; 46,368; 75,025; 121,393; 196,418; 317,811; 514,229; 832,040; 1,346,269; 2,178,309...and on into infinity. Each number is the sum of the two preceding numbers, and the series can extend indefinitely.

The most apparent link with nature is the frequency with which these numbers occur in plants and in animals. Octopuses and spiders have eight legs; starfish have five points. Tree branches and pine needles tend to cluster in groups of two, three, or five. The famous four-leaf clover is a rarity among the predominantly three-leaf versions. Petunias have 5 leaves, schefflera have mostly 8, black-eyed Susans have 21, and daisies have 34 and 55.

And the pattern continues: There are 13 stripes on a ringtailed lemur, 13 stripes on a striped ground squirrel. Sunflower seeds flow from the center of the head in logarithmic or ever-expanding spirals, generally having 21, 34, 55, 89, or even 144 seeds. Even the way a plant grows and spreads out its leaves most often reflects an exact Fibonacci number or pattern.

But even more intriguing, and what fascinated Fibonacci, is a *remarkable relationship between the numbers,* called the golden ratio.

Fibonacci Rabbits

Here's Fibonacci's puzzle: If an adult pair of rabbits produced another pair every month, and each new pair began reproducing when it was two months old, how many rabbits would be born each month?

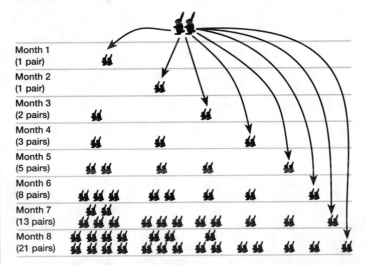

Month 1
(1 pair)

Month 2
(1 pair)

Month 3
(2 pairs)

Month 4
(3 pairs)

Month 5
(5 pairs)

Month 6
(8 pairs)

Month 7
(13 pairs)

Month 8
(21 pairs)

Count 'em: The number of pairs of newborn rabbits each successive month is 1, 1, 2, 3, 5, 8, 13, and so on. By the eighth month, you're up to 21 pairs...and every month there are more and more baby rabbits born. The number of rabbits born each month is always the sum of the preceding two numbers. Thirteen is the sum of 8 and 5; 21 is the sum of 13 and 8; and so on.

A Pleasing Proportion

The golden ratio—also called the golden proportion—is found by dividing each Fibonacci number, after the first few, by the number that follows it. The answer always approximates

(continued on page 20)

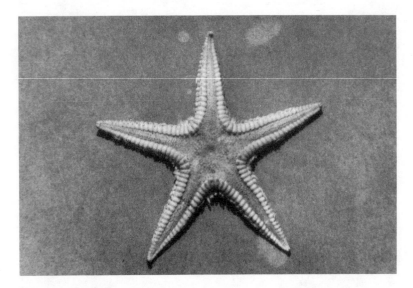

Starfish—5 points

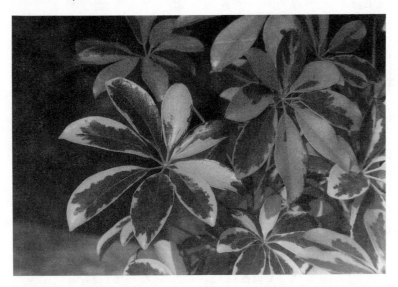

Schefflera—clusters of 8 leaves

Nature's Pattern: Fibonacci numbers abound in nature, in the number of petals, leaves or flowers on plants, and even the number of ridges on shells.

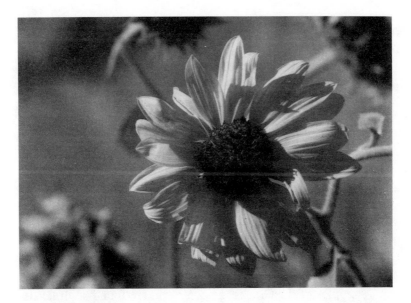

Daisy—21 petals

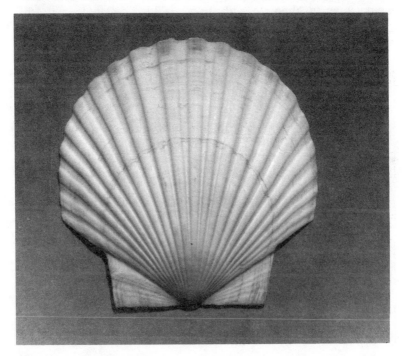

Shell—21 ridges

0.618. After 144, the first three numbers in the decimal are always 0.618. Actually, the divisions approach 0.618034 but never exactly reach it. This result or mathematical function is known as phi, and the ratio of 0.618:1 as the golden ratio.

Dividing any number in the sequence by the preceding number approximates another number, 1.618.

Researchers have found evidence of the golden proportion of 0.618:1 and the proportion of 1.618:1 as far back as ancient Egypt and Greece. Although it is uncertain how much of the precise mathematics the Greeks knew, they used what they called the golden mean throughout their art and architecture. They defined the golden mean as the point that divides a line into two parts so the smaller part is in the same proportion to the larger part as the larger part is to the entire line. That proportion always equals 0.618:1.

Examples of the Greeks' golden mean are found at all levels of their works. Before the Parthenon began to fall into ruin, it would have fit almost exactly into a golden rectangle, with the

THE GOLDEN MEAN

The golden mean is the point that divides a line so that the proportion of the smaller part of the line (*a* in the diagram below) to the larger part of the line (*b*) is the same as the proportion of that larger part (*b*) to the whole line (*c*). And here's the connection to Fibonacci numbers: The proportion of those lines to each other is 0.618:1—the golden ratio, the same ratio each Fibonacci number has to the one following it.

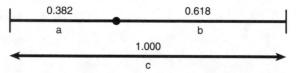

When **a:b** equals **b:c**, the point between **a** and **b** is the golden mean.

sides of the rectangle in 0.618:1 proportions. Greek sculpture of the human body is based on the navel as the golden mean of the body, with the distance from the feet to the navel measuring 0.618 of the length of the whole body. The upper portion was then divided again in golden proportion at the neck and eyes. One famous Greek sculptor, Phidias, was so attached to the concept that all of his figures were carved in detailed golden proportion.

The Greeks relied on the golden mean because they believed it was the most pleasing proportion to the human eye. They strove for balance and harmony in art, architecture, mind, and body. The golden mean reflected the epitome of balance and harmony in their material world, and history has supported its allure: Greek architecture, sculpture, and craftswork are still considered the quintessence of beauty, the most pleasing of all artwork to behold.

Throughout recorded history, other examples of the golden ratio appear. The ancient Egyptians were well aware of it, and the Great Pyramids as well as the triangles, pentagons, and pentagrams inscribed on their inner walls are all astonishing displays of the golden mean. Remarkably, the Hebrew Ark of the Covenant was built in the same 0.618:1 proportion.

Leonardo da Vinci used the golden ratio in his paintings and sculpture, even coauthoring a book about it, *De Devina Proportione*. Michelangelo's famous sixteenth-century sculpture *David* is another example of this ancient beauty. Fibonacci's proportions, so pleasing to the eye that they have been taught in art schools, were used by many other great artists, from Bellini to Poussin to Seurat.

Spirals of Gold

As time went on, more was discovered about the "magic" of the golden proportion. For example, a golden rectangle is defined as having a width that is 0.618 of the length. When a square is created within the golden rectangle as shown on page 22, the result is a secondary rectangle with its sides in exactly the same proportion as the original—0.618:1.

(continued on page 24)

EVOLVING GOLDEN SPIRALS

If you drew a square in a golden rectangle, you'd be left with another, smaller golden rectangle. If you drew a square in that golden rectangle you'd get—you guessed it—another, smaller golden rectangle. If you drew as many squares as possible and then connected the centers of all the squares, you'd get a golden spiral.

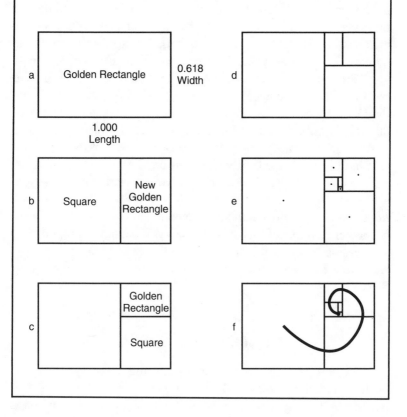

GOLDEN SPIRAL

This shape, so pervasive in nature, has very specific proportions. If you draw any diameter through the center *x* as shown, the longer part of that line (from *a* to *x*) is 0.618 of the whole line (*a* to *d*). This proportion holds true within each curve of the spiral: *b* to *x* would be 0.618 of the distance from *b* to *c*, and so on as the spiral gets smaller.

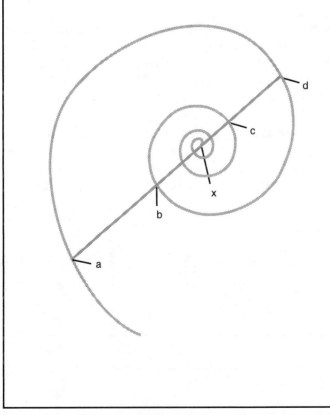

If you divide that rectangle into a square, another square and another golden rectangle are formed. Mathematicians have found that continuing this pattern and then connecting the centers of all the squares will result in a specific swirl whose geometric properties adhere precisely to the golden ratio of 0.618034:1. Scientists have named these precise swirls "logarithmic" or "golden" spirals, and it's amazing how often you can find them in nature.

The nautilus shell, which extends as the animal inside grows, forms a golden spiral as it develops. The same spiral can be found in other seashells, ram horns, elephant tusks, flowers and plant growth patterns, scorpion tails, pineapples—even the double spiral of the DNA molecule, the part of our chromosomes that carries our genetic material.

Most horns, claws, and teeth throughout the animal kingdom grow along the path of the golden spiral. It is especially obvious in ram horns and parrot beaks, and only slightly less so in elephant tusks and lion claws. There is even evidence of the spiral as far back as the saber-toothed tiger and the mammoth. It also shows up in 350-million-year-old mollusk shells.

But the spiral is found well beyond the limits of living organisms. Ocean wave curls that are so dear to surfers are beautiful displays of golden spirals in motion. Comet tails, hurricanes, the orbital pathways of subatomic particles, and spiral galaxies of

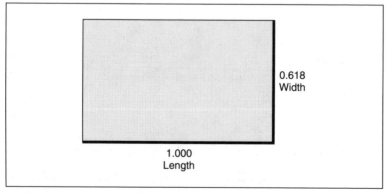

0.618
Width

1.000
Length

Golden Rectangle: *A golden rectangle is one whose sides are in a 0.618:1 proportion to each other.*

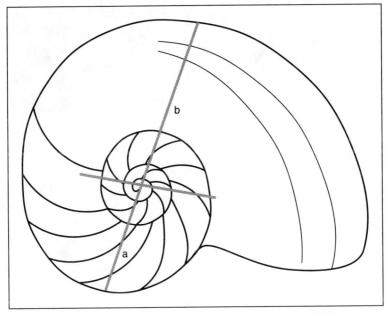

Spiral in a Shell: _A nautilus shell forms a perfect golden spiral—line_ **a** _is 0.618 of line_ **b**, _and line_ **b** _is 0.618 of_ **a** _plus_ **b**.

stars demonstrate that this pattern and proportion have existed for billions upon billions of years. The proportion scientists now refer to as "nature's way" is also the path of least resistance.

The golden spiral seems to have no limit as to size. As the spiral appears in our DNA, the distance between the coils that form the spiral are so tiny that the distance between them measures about 35 angstroms. (There are 250 million angstroms to an inch.) But the same spiral can also be seen in formations as huge as galaxies of stars that are 100,000 light-years in diameter. (One light-year is 5.88 trillion miles.)

Golden Proportions within Us

The human body is also arranged along the principles of the Fibonacci numbers and spirals. We each have five extensions from our trunk—two arms, two legs, and a head. There are five lobes

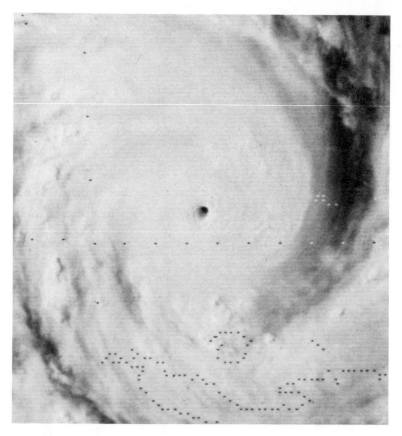

Destructive Spirals: Some golden spirals occur in destructive forms--such as Hurricane Gilbert.

to our lungs, three on the right side, two on the left. The branches of our bronchial tree have short and long tubes that are approximately in a 0.618:1 proportion. The fiber arrangement in the muscles of our hearts and the formation of parts of our brains all approximate golden spirals.

The "coincidence" goes still deeper. Even the fetal position is representative of a golden spiral. (See the photograph on page 29.)

And just as our DNA molecule spirals in this proportion, so does the rotating movement of our muscles when contracted. Nautilus machines are designed to take advantage of that spiral,

ORDER OUT OF CHAOS

The rise and fall of stock market prices. Weather fluctuations. The shape of our bronchial tree. The number of petals on a flower. The patterns in our DNA. It's hard to imagine a connection among this varied collection. At first glance, these behaviors and shapes appear random or chaotic, and certainly unrelated.

What all these things have in common, however, is that beneath the apparent chaos lurks a definite and definable order. In many cases, this order can be described by Fibonacci numbers, the Chaos theory, fractal geometry, or a combination of the three.

Chaos theory, popularized by James Gleick in his book _Chaos: Making a New Science_ in 1987, unveils certain patterns in apparently chaotic occurrences. Patterns are evident in air currents, heat currents, population explosions, and even epidemics. Fractals, described by Benoit Mandelbrot in his 1982 book _The Fractal Geometry of Nature,_ are identical shapes or patterns in varying scales. Each fluctuation or shape within the fractal system is of the same pattern, but on a different scale. This can be seen in market price fluctuations or the shape of our lungs, a coral formation, clouds, and coastlines.

Fibonacci numbers, as you learn in this chapter, are a series of numbers, all with a nearly identical proportion to each other. This proportion is evident in many natural forms: shells, tornadoes, ocean waves, some of our body parts, and even our DNA.

The laws and proportions of chaos, fractals, and Fibonacci numbers all make evident a thread of commonality between many diverse systems and occurrences. You could think of these patterns as simply being nature's way: the path of least resistance. While the origin and nature of "chaotic" behavior are far from clear-cut, a close look at some of these apparently irregular or erratic natural patterns reveals at least a peek at some of the secrets of nature, and a chance to use them to our benefit.

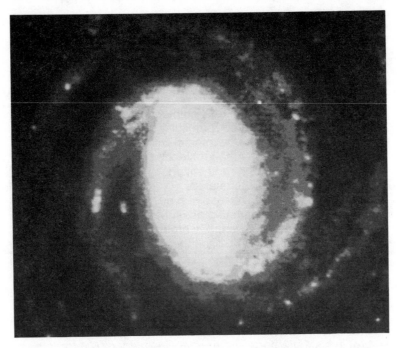

Whirling Galaxy: You can easily see the spiral shape in galaxy NGC 1232, a galaxy in the constellation of Eridanus. Many similar galaxies contain billions of stars that form enormous spirals.

exercising muscles in what approximates the body's most natural movement. The founder of Aikido, Morihei Uyeshiba, incorporated the spiral pattern into his martial art system. He frequently observed, "The movement of Aikido is the movement of Nature—whose secret is profound and infinite."

The most intricate of pleasures also relate to Fibonacci numbers. Music, for example, is based on an eight-note octave—on a piano represented by five black keys and eight white keys. The major sixth, the musical interval that's the most pleasing to us, has frequencies that are in a ratio of 8:5. That's a proportion of 0.62500:1, quite close to the golden ratio.

This sound is heard by the cochlea of the inner ear—yet another of our organs that is shaped in a golden spiral. So you're listening to Fibonacci-structured musical sounds with your Fibonacci-structured inner ear.

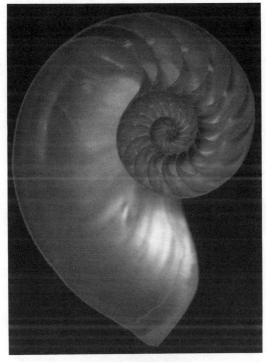

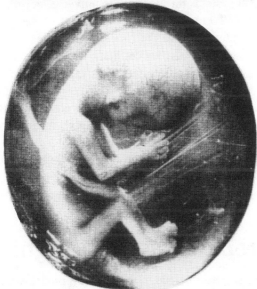

Spirals in Humans and Animals: The human fetus evolves in a shape similar to the golden spiral, seen clearly in the nautilus shell.

CHAPTER FOUR

TRANSLATING SCIENCE TO HUMAN PERFORMANCE

So how do Fibonacci numbers apply to training performances? The pattern described by Fibonacci numbers, evident in so many natural systems throughout the universe, occurs in human energies as well. To understand and make use of the connection, you need to be familiar with the Elliott Wave Principle.

Ralph Nelson Elliott, an accountant in the early 1900s, specialized in railroad and restaurant management. He had a keen mind for detail and a flair for long, laborious mathematical analyses. His book, *Tea Room and Cafeteria Management,* showcased not only his expertise in restaurant management and accounting but also his rigorous and exacting attention to detail.

This obsession with detail and clarity allowed Elliott to plot the supposedly unplottable—man's psychological response to free will, as it occurs in the stock market.

From Illness to Insight

Elliott's expertise in accounting and corporate reorganization took him all over the world, working for several organizations. His last position, as general auditor of the International Railways of Guatemala, ended with a serious illness that required a long recuperation. But during these years of forced inactivity, Elliott turned his attention to studying data that would form the basis for the Elliott Wave Principle.

Working from a chair on his front porch, Elliott pored over hundreds of stock market fluctuations. He found yearly, monthly, weekly, and daily records going back 75 years, and constructed his own hourly and half-hourly graphs by using Dow charts and the tapes off the floor of a brokerage house. Elliott became as obsessed with analyzing the ebb and flow of the market as he had been with his earlier occupations. When he finished his research, he had discovered an order to the behavior of the market that corresponds to a blueprint of human response and performance.

Wave after Wave

Elliott discovered that human behavior, as illustrated by the exercise of free will in the stock market, can be graphed as a series of waves within waves that conform mathematically to Fibonacci's sequence of numbers. The stock marketplace is a large-scale example of the results of free will, as everyone involved is free to choose when and what to buy and sell.

The Elliott Wave is comprised of a five- and three-wave cycle, which then repeats and expands. For every five movements or waves upward, there are three movements down, for a total of eight actions. Remember that three, five, and eight are all Fibonacci numbers? Still more Fibonacci numbers appear when the cycle is expanded. Each movement or "wave" upward, which represents each rise in the market, is "corrected" by a corresponding wave downward, or market depression.

According to Elliott's theory, the stock market never actually crashes, but merely corrects a previous advance so it can advance to a new high. People who are unaware of the nature of the advancing wave are dismayed by the downward correction, while those who are aware of the patterns know that the next phase will be an upward one. Since there are always more upward than

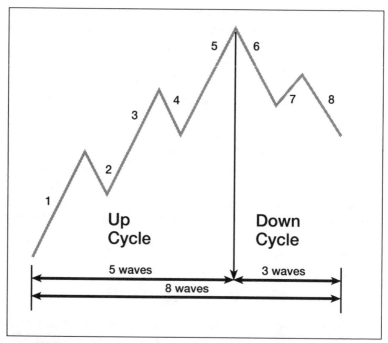

The Elliott Wave: *The basic Elliott Wave has an up cycle and a down cycle. In the up cycle, there are three waves or movements up and two down, and in the down cycle there are two down waves and one up wave. This cycle repeats indefinitely.*

Adapted from Prechter and Frost, *Elliott Wave Principle,* 1985.

downward movements, the result in the long run is an infinite progression in the marketplace.

Within each wave in the cycle is a series of smaller waves: Each of the individual upward movements is comprised of three small upward and two small downward movements. Each downward wave is comprised of two smaller downward and one smaller upward movement (see ''The Elliott Wave'' illustration above). As with the Fibonacci numbers, the Elliott Wave is a never-ending sequence.

Investors who want a better grasp on their portfolios can read *Elliott Wave Principle* by Alfred Frost and Robert Prechter and

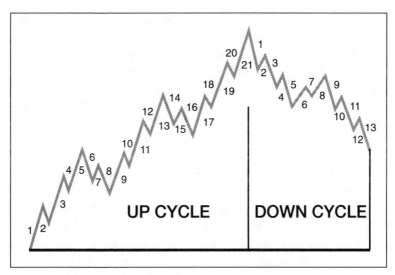

The Complete Cycle: _Each upward wave or movement in the Elliott Wave breaks down into other, smaller advances and regressions. Notice the occurrences of Fibonacci numbers: Each peak in the up cycle has five waves in the upward movement and three in the downward movement, for a total of eight. There are 21 waves in this expanded up cycle and 13 in the expanded down cycle, for a total of 34._

Adapted from diagram by Robert Prechter.

The Major Works of R. N. Elliott by Robert Prechter. However, for the purposes of sports or personal performance, what you need to understand about the Elliott Wave is that generally low points are followed by high points, even higher than the previous high, and that the cycle of highs and lows repeats in a specific pattern.

Math Agrees with Philosophy

Elliott's mathematical discovery was hardly a new concept. Danish philosopher and theologian Søren Kierkegaard, one of the founders of modern existentialism, said there must be a major reversal or shock to lead to any kind of progress, whether the progress of humanity or the progress of the individual. His theory was that something decisive always occurs by a jerk or a sudden turn. These progress-inducing reversals, shocks, or turns—called "evolutionary drivers" by some anthropologists—occur in animals when evolution forces major changes in a species.

On both a large and small scale it becomes evident that low points precede high points. Because highs and lows are progressively cyclic, the reverse is also true: A peak comes before a valley, a high precedes a low.

The Elliott Wave Principle illustrates the one-step-back and two-steps-forward philosophy, a way of thought that has been endorsed by many other great thinkers. What Kierkegaard refers to as high points, Elliott calls advancing waves; what Kierkegaard describes as a low, Elliott points out is actually a constructive correction. Both doctrines agree that the downward turn is necessary to give impetus to the upward swing.

The Athletic Connection

Athletes regularly encounter advancements and corrections or highs and lows in their performances. Do you know who once held the record for the most strikeouts of any major league baseball player? It was Babe Ruth, the home run *and* strikeout king of his time. He tallied a career 1,330 strikeouts to accompany his record 714 home runs. Mickey Mantle, also known for his great hitting ability and his 536 home runs, held another record with 1,710 strikeouts. The current strikeout champ is Reggie Jackson with 2,597 strikeouts—but Jackson is better remembered for his 563 homers.

Just as the ups and downs of the Elliott Wave Principle can be expanded or contracted to apply to both larger and smaller phenomena, so can the home run/strikeout phenomenon in sports. On a larger scale, looking at teams rather than individuals, the Detroit Tigers in 1991 led all 26 major league baseball teams with the most home runs *and* the most strikeouts.

As an individual or a team progresses, they reach higher peaks but also have deeper valleys. When the peaks and valleys occur is controllable with intelligent training—and *that's what Consistent Winning is all about.*

Highs and lows occur as naturally in an athlete's performance as elsewhere in life. The orbit of the moon, the pull of the tides, the life of a love affair all share the common rhythm of high and low, give and take, push and pull, mountain and valley, yin and yang. So the question develops: How can an athlete control the flow and timing of these tides, minimizing the negative of the lows, the valleys, while at the same time maximizing the positive of the highs, the peaks?

Taking Control of Your Cycles

In summary, the Elliott Wave transforms Fibonacci numbers and their proportion into a graph depicting advancements and corrections. As you have seen in chapter 3, we as humans fit the golden proportion physically. We also fit it physiologically. This proportion will be more evident after you have read chapters 7, 8, and 9, which describe the Consistent Winning cycles. For our purposes, we can correlate the advancements or upward movements to training periods, and the corrections or downward movements to resting periods—or, if resting periods are not taken, to periods when you are prone to illness or injury.

Once it was established from athletes' records that the peaks of their performances correspond naturally to the crest of the ascending wave of the Elliott Wave Principle, it was apparent that most injuries and "off" days must occur during the low points or "correcting" waves.

The answer to taking control became obvious: Instead of continuing to train during these low points, you must *rest, or reduce training.*

The important point is that you can manipulate the cycle of ups and downs. You don't just hope that your performance occurs during an upward wave. You *choose* your own low and high points: In essence you create a controlled "low" by resting at a specific time. And because low points in performances are followed by high points at certain definite intervals, you're also creating a controlled "high"—exactly when you want it.

THE UPS AND DOWNS OF ATHLETIC PERFORMANCE

Here's how your performances fit into the Elliott Wave—and how you can schedule "high" performances. The upward waves or movements represent training, and the downward waves represent resting. By scheduling your rest periods at specific times, you start the cycle that will end with a peak performance a certain number of days later.

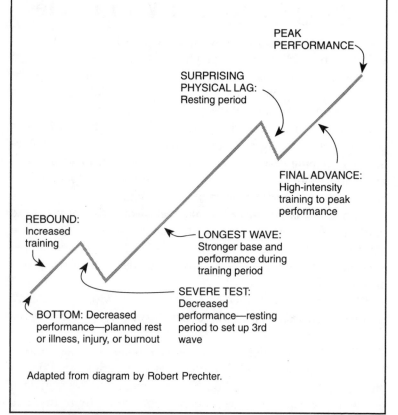

PEAK
PERFORMANCE

SURPRISING
PHYSICAL LAG:
Resting period

FINAL ADVANCE:
High-intensity
training to peak
performance

REBOUND:
Increased
training

LONGEST WAVE:
Stronger base and
performance during
training period

SEVERE TEST:
Decreased
performance—resting
period to set up 3rd
wave

BOTTOM: Decreased
performance—planned rest
or illness, injury, or burnout

Adapted from diagram by Robert Prechter.

CHAPTER FIVE

REST: YOU NEED IT TO EXCEL

Athletes, in general, don't like to rest. Lyn Brooks, now a dedicated user of Consistent Winning, originally resisted the idea of rest. Before trying the system, she declared, "If I take a week off, I'm afraid I'll lose everything!"

This idea, held by casual amateur and ardent professional alike, is a misconception. Rest, forced on a performer from illness or injury, has preceded many world records and other great performances. There are numerous examples of athletes excelling after enforced rests, such as Katrin Doerre's 1987 marathon win and Mary Decker Slaney's standout 3,000-meter win in 1988.

Katrin Doerre of East Germany won the Tokyo International Women's Marathon by more than a minute on November 15, 1987, with a time of 2:25:24. Because of a leg injury she'd suffered in June, Doerre told reporters, "At first I never expected to win . . . but the three-month rest produced my best time!"

Mary Decker Slaney, a world-class runner, missed most of the 1987 running season because of an Achilles tendon injury. She set a 1988 U.S. best while winning the women's 3,000-meter race in the Bruce Jenner Track and Field Classic. She reported that she felt better than she had in years.

Your Training Base Has Staying Power

Every athlete, musician, artist, and other performer regularly relies on the reserves built up over months and years of effort, whether physical or mental. This reserve, known as the "training base," cannot be erased or disengaged by a few days of inactivity—or even 21 days of inactivity!

Maximal exercise measures—which include VO_2 max, maximal heart rate, maximal speed, and workload—are maintained for 10 to 28 days with training reductions of 70 to 80 percent, according to exercise physiologist Joseph A. Houmard, Ph.D., of the Human Performance Laboratory at East Carolina University in South Carolina. And muscular power is maintained *or improved* with a 60 to 90 percent reduction in training for 6 to 21 days, he says. "Endurance athletes should not refrain from reduced training prior to competition in an effort to improve performance," states Dr. Houmard.

Research at Ball State University in Muncie, Indiana, showed that aerobic capacity in swimmers with a good training base was retained during four weeks while they trained only one day a week. Aerobic conditioning effects were not lost until *six to eight weeks* after regular training ceased.

Consistent Winning, however, at no time advocates taking more than two days of total rest in a row. Resting periods are punctuated with active rest days, during which you do light exercise. Long rests that provide a rest base for the 3-Month Cycle include not only active rest days but also easy- to moderate-exercise days. Putting yourself through the physical and mental stress of "exercise withdrawal" to take advantage of this natural cycle is never necessary.

The key to overcoming your fear of taking time off is to understand how much it will help, rather than hinder, your performance. You need to know about these elements of Consistent Winning.

- What naturally occurring cycles are

- When they take place
- What the catapult effect is and why it works
- How you can control your own cycles to achieve pre-scheduled peak performances, whenever you want them

After many successes with Consistent Winning, Lyn Brooks now actually looks forward to her rest days. "I know they're going to help me," she says. Rest days will help you, too. The secret to controlling your own peak performance is knowing *when* and *how long* to rest. Properly timed resting creates the key element of Consistent Winning—the "catapult effect."

Catapult Your Efforts

A catapult is set by pulling it backward: The backward movement creates a potential for a powerful force, ready to be released when the catapult is sprung.

Resting at a specific time has this exact effect—and for that reason we call it the catapult effect. You can control and focus this powerful potential force of all your accumulated training by pulling back or resting at the correct time in your own Consistent Winning schedule.

Resting at the appropriate times allows your body to recover, rebuild, and become stronger. It also *creates* the downward movement of your personal Elliott Wave cycle. Remember that in the Elliott Wave, after a downward movement comes an upward one, to an even higher level. In the case of sports, that higher level translates to a peak performance.

Your resting period acts as a catapult to maximum performance. You have in essence created a valley that propels you onward to a new and higher peak. "Detraining"—allowing your body to recover from training by resting—at the correct time is an essential part of training to achieve greater performances.

No training system can guarantee you will perform well. However, Consistent Winning does increase the chances that you will have the edge to perform at your best.

PHYSICAL OVERUSE CAN EQUAL ABUSE

A great benefit of the regular resting periods built into Consistent Winning is that they keep you from exercising *too much.* Athletes—even amateurs—need to remember that training for maximum performance is not synonymous with physical abuse. Regular exercise is a great habit—but at safe dosage levels.

To a certain point, being addicted to exercise can be positive. But it can become destructive when your training cycles do not include resting periods. Exercise addiction can destroy your ability to cope with or gain satisfaction from anything else in life except training.

Continued training without resting days leads to abnormal tolerance of the workload—you're no longer able to recognize signals from your body that it's time to stop. You may feel you need to *increase* your training when what you really need is recovery and rest. At this point, training doesn't lead to improvement but can actually damage your body.

Physical signs of addiction may include excess loss of body weight, loss of sleep, constant soreness and stiffness, decreased appetite, loss of vigor, decreased sexual drive, increased resting heart rate, and increased blood pressure. The high levels of stress can suppress the immune system, and you may become sick more often and more seriously than nonathletes. Continuing to overtrain may lead to physical breakdown, exhaustion, and burnout.

Be careful, though. If you *abruptly* cease exercise after overtraining, you may have withdrawal symptoms that can include irritability, anxiety, poor concentration, sleep disturbances, and depression. You may even feel guilty and experience a drop in self-esteem from missing a workout and feel compelled to exercise harder the next day to make up for it.

The solution is to allow regular resting periods. This helps you have high resilience to stress in general and good self-esteem. Your body will function at peak efficiency, and even your immune system will likely be strengthened by this healthy range of training.

Maximal Improveme in 12 Weeks

The catapult effect can also be seen in laboratory results that measure mitochondrial activity. (Mitochondria are the parts of muscle cells that make energy for work.) Studies have shown that when a person begins training from a rested or slightly detrained condition, the activity of cytochrome c, which is a mitochondrial enzyme involved in energy production, begins to build. So does the maximum amount of oxygen the body uses, which is known as VO_2 max. After 12 weeks of training following a rest, cytochrome c reaches its peak and then begins to drop.

At this point the body must be allowed to rest and regroup for continued progress. Continued training beyond 12 weeks will only result in a drop of both cytochrome c activity and VO_2 max, and hence a drop in performance.

In a study at the Wellington Clinical School of Medicine in Wellington, New Zealand, weekly running distances for six male subjects were increased from 20 kilometers per week to 73 kilometers per week over a period of 36 weeks while training for a marathon. The runners' anaerobic threshold—the maximum effort they could put forth without getting out of breath—increased signficantly during the first 12 weeks of training. It didn't rise thereafter for the next 24 weeks. Their VO_2 max, or maximal oxygen uptake, also increased the most in the first 12 weeks of training. It increased only slightly more in the second 12 weeks, and not at all in the final 12 weeks.

Avoiding Excessive Overload

Training can be described as stressing or overloading any of the body's systems so they become better or stronger. This is called the overload principle and involves pushing the systems to do more than they have done before. These systems include muscles, bones, heart, lungs, glands, lymph, blood, connective tissue, and nervous system. The positive effect of overloading is obvious

WHY VO₂ MAX IS IMPORTANT

Maximal oxygen uptake, or VO_2 max, is widely used as a measure of aerobic fitness. The V represents the volume of gas taken up by the body over time, in this case oxygen (O_2). Because the muscles have to use oxygen in order to function, measuring how much oxygen the body uses in a given time provides a way to measure how efficiently the body is working. The *max* represents the maximum amount of work that can be done during high-intensity exercise.

This effort is measured during exercise on a treadmill or stationary bicycle so work intensity can be carefully controlled. Samples of air from the exercising person are monitored for volume and concentration of oxygen. The harder the person is working, the more oxygen will be picked up by the body and used in the working muscles. (The VO_2 is measured in units of milliliters of oxygen per kilogram of total body weight per minute.)

The muscles use oxygen to burn fuel—mostly fats, but also carbohydrates and a little protein—to release energy for movement, body heat, and other biochemical processes. This chemical burning process is known as aerobic metabolism.

VO_2 max is very low in people who don't exercise much and is high in people who do regular aerobic exercise. Therefore, VO_2 max is widely used as a measure of aerobic fitness. The American College of Sports Medicine has established ranges of VO_2 max for different levels of aerobic fitness.

MAXIMAL OXYGEN UPTAKE LEVELS

Level of Aerobic Fitness	VO₂ max* (ml/kg/min)
High	49.0–56.0
Good	39.0–48.9
Average	25.0–38.9
Low	14.0–24.9
Poor	3.5–13.9

* For 40-year-old males.

in weight lifting: Muscles noticeably increase in size and strength. The overload principle holds true for other types of exercise, including endurance training. In contrast, underloading causes noticeable decreases in size and strength of the body's systems.

Endurance training, which causes changes in muscle, may be destructive. Cell mitochondria swell, metabolic wastes accumulate, essential nutrients (such as electrolytes and glycogen) deplete, and muscle tissue is torn. This tearing is known as microtrauma of the cells, and torn muscle tissue does not work efficiently. Muscles take about 48 hours to recover from this process. Balanced training, however, keeps the destruction to a level that gives tissues time for adequate recovery so they are stronger and work more efficiently than before. Alternating easy and hard workouts according to your Consistent Winning schedule is important because it helps balance the breakdown and rebuilding cycle.

If your body doesn't complete the rebuilding phase, conditioning slows down, and your body does not recover or make the most of training. In some cases of overtraining, the building and conditioning process can cease or even reverse. For example, one study found that the thigh circumferences of overtrained bicycle racers actually decreased while they were still active. Heavy overuse induced muscle atrophy and actually hindered performance.

In order to see steady improvement, you must establish a balance between overuse (too much stress) and underuse (too little stress). This balance is maintained by alternating periods of training with planned periods of rest. As cycles of resting and training accumulate, you build a training base, and the body systems you are training recover more quickly and become stronger than they were before. Balancing of rest and training leads to maximum improvement. You help maintain this balance by alternating easy and hard training days and by taking extra rest days whenever needed.

Ultramarathoner Nick Bassett, who regularly runs 50-plus-mile races, remarks, "Out of my whole training schedule, the toughest thing is to rest, but I know I have to do it. You need to be a physical animal to run ultramarathons, but you need to be a 'mental animal' to rest."

CHAPTER SIX

WHY YOU WIN WITH CONSISTENT WINNING

Consistent Winning is not a method of drill, a schedule of repeated exercise, or any other intrusion into your own program of workout and/or training. It is a timing cycle that restructures your personal schedule of when and how long to rest and train. The rest/train ratios are in tune with the natural patterns of valleys and peaks inherent in the golden proportion explained in chapter 3. You control the timing of the Consistent Winning cycles.

Choose Your Cycles

To control the timing of your own peak performance you must first adjust your schedule to include a Consistent Winning cycle. There are three basic cycles—3-Day Cycle, 3-Week Cycle, and 3-Month Cycle—which can be used either alone or together.

Here's how the cycles are set up.

3-Day Cycle: A three-day resting period (an easy day and two resting days) followed by three training days. The peak performance is on day 3 of training.

BEGINNERS CAN BENEFIT, TOO

Les Gottlieb of Huntington Beach, California, noticed that his weight was creeping up by about a pound a year. Then at a health screening in the local mall, he discovered that his cholesterol levels were uncomfortably high.

Soon thereafter Gottlieb read an article suggesting walking to burn off calories and help lose weight. So he began to walk.

If Gottlieb were like most people who begin exercise programs, after about three weeks of his new regimen he would have quit. But he didn't. Instead, he continued to walk, lost weight, and even added bicycling, joined a gym, and lengthened his walks.

What were Gottlieb's secrets for success?

There were several. First, he was determined, and he made a commitment to an exercise program. For most of us, that's good for a week or two. Second, Gottlieb started *slowly* and built up *gradually*. He used the timing in the Consistent Winning cycles to train and rest appropriately, and that helped him avoid injury and pain.

Finally, Gottlieb got past that magic three-week point. According to psychologists, it takes three weeks to form a habit. And according to the Consistent Winning technique, you reach a peak after three weeks of training—which is followed by a downturn, or period of lesser performance, both physically and mentally. Gottlieb was aware that this disappointing period would occur, and he looked past it.

There are three keys that people beginning an exercise program should keep in mind: commitment, gradual progression, and forming a habit. If you remember these and adhere to the resting cycles built into Consistent Winning, you'll find it easier to incorporate regular exercise into your life.

3-Week Cycle: A five-day resting period (four resting days with a training day in the middle) followed by 21 training days. The peak day is training day 21.

3-Month Cycle: A 13-day resting period (don't worry, there are five training days in there) followed by 12 weeks of training to peak performance.

Each cycle works by itself and can be used individually. However, when the cycles are used together and superimposed on one another in an overlapping structure, they are set to end together on the same day, producing a more powerful effect. Using this overlap structure, resting periods appear naturally at the junctures between the cycles, in essence forming the downward or correcting wave that catapults the upward cycle.

After the right amount of rest, you will peak after three months, three weeks, and/or three days of training. The resting

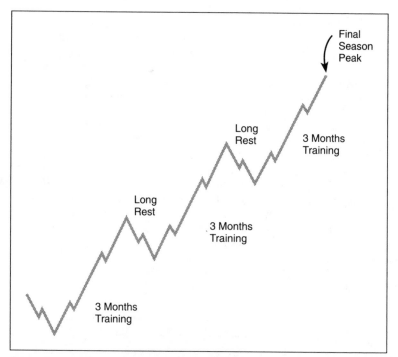

Climbing to Higher Performances: *Consistent Winning cycles build on each other, leading to higher and higher performance peaks. This depicts three 3-Month Cycles, one after the other. During the up waves, you're training; during the down waves, you're resting. These resting periods form the "catapult" for the next up wave.*

periods scheduled before the three months, three weeks, or three days of training will set up peak performance on the last day of these training periods.

What Exactly Does Resting Mean?

Before we get into the cycles, you should know what we consider to be rest. There are two types of rest days: active rest days, when you do very easy and limited activity, and rest days, when you completely avoid any workout greater than a 30-minute walk.

A resting period need never have more than two rest days in a row without a workout. All short resting periods include one or more active rest days, while long resting periods also include light exercise days. *The last two days in any resting period must be rest days to set up the training cycle peaks.*

The exception to this rule is the Monday/Thursday resting schedule used for consecutive Saturday events, which is explained in chapter 11.

Active Rest. Active rest days allow for a maximum of 20 to 30 minutes of light training. Twenty minutes of training acts as physical therapy for your muscles and joints. It is enough time to break into a sweat, keep the body and psyche ''well oiled,'' allow healing, and avoid fear of losing your physical edge, but not enough time for your body to actually gear up. Thirty minutes of aerobic training can achieve maximum heart efficiency without crossing the line between active rest and destructive training from which the body will rebound, causing a training effect.

A general rule of thumb is to keep active rest at one-third of the duration of your regular training, and at a lower intensity. For example, a marathoner who habitually runs 1 to 1½ hours a day might put in 20 to 30 minutes at an easy pace on an active rest day.

Rest. Rest days mean just that: no training. That means no running, weight lifting, or body stressing related to your sports.

To prevent psychological withdrawal symptoms and to keep your body and psyche lubricated, a 20- to 30-minute moderately paced walk is advisable. Too fast a walk will create an aerobic training effect. A moderate walk should be below 50 percent of your maximum aerobic capacity. Exercise intensity can be gauged by heart rate—your approximate maximal heart rate equals 220 minus your age. During your walk, check your pulse to ensure that your heart rate doesn't exceed half of your maximal heart rate.

Blueprint for Human Performance

Each of the three Consistent Winning cycles is complete by itself and can be used individually. When the cycles are used together, however, they are superimposed onto each other so that the final day of each cycle is the same day: your event day, the day you want to peak. Whether you use one, two, or all three of the cycles depends on how far in the future your event is and the complexity of your schedule.

To determine which cycle to use for your next event or desired peak, count backward from your desired maximum performance day. The shortest effective cycle (3-Day) begins with a resting period five days prior to the maximum performance day. The longest single cycle (3-Month) requires a 13-day resting period beginning 96 days in advance of your maximum performance day. There are many minor peaks throughout the ideal schedule. For example, after every resting period there is a peak three days later.

It is important that you return to training very slowly after a resting period or time away from training for any reason. A gradual increase in the amount and intensity of your training is paramount to your well-being and the success of the technique. If you push too hard during training (overtrain), you risk decreasing the strength of your peak performance, and you may get hurt.

Because Consistent Winning is based on a recurring natural phenomenon that allows for some variety, adjustments and minor

PLANNING
HUMAN PERFORMANCE

A 3-Month Cycle also incorporates a 3-Day
a 3-Week Cycle, combining them so they all end
same day. (You can use the shorter cycles separat   ut
when combined they produce a greater peak effect.) Notice
the Fibonacci numbers: The number of weeks in each
training period are 3, 5, and 3. The number of days in each
training period are 21, 34, 15, and 3, and the resting
periods themselves are made up of 13, 3, 5, and 3 days.

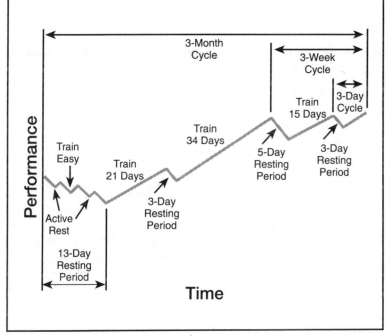

deviations may be made in the resting periods once you have a
solid training base. For example, if you were scheduled for a five-
day rest, you could begin your resting period earlier and take as

...n as a week off, as long as you still trained the requisite number of days.

The training periods are fixed in that you should begin and end them as scheduled, although you *can* insert unscheduled rest days if you become tired or are unable to train for other reasons. Keep deviations to a minimum, and try to have two rest days immediately before beginning a training period to ensure setting up the exact peak day.

Because there are three cycles of different lengths, the Consistent Winning technique can be adapted to the entire season's schedule. The exact timing of the cycles and how to use them is explained in the chapters that follow.

TENDENCY, NOT A LAW

For the athletes studied during the development and testing of the Consistent Winning technique—and for both authors, who use the cycles for their own athletic endeavors—Consistent Winning has held true at least 80 percent of the time. Better than four out of five times, a peak performance occurred when expected, despite occasionally losing track of cycles or missing four, five, or as many as seven days of training in a row.

On the other hand, less than 20 percent of the time, a "peak day" that's due does not appear. Outside circumstances, such as accidents or personal emergencies, can occur. The day that was supposed to be a peak day will be a good day, but not a wonder-where-it-came-from day. But even in nature the Fibonacci sequence is not an absolute law; it's a strong natural tendency. The Fibonacci phenomenon appears in nature not quite often enough to be absolute, but too often to be discounted or ignored. This is why this technique is called *Consistent* Winning rather than *Absolute* Winning.

CHAPTER SEVEN

THE 3-DAY CYCLE: TO PEAK NEXT WEEK

The 3-Day Cycle of Consistent Winning, the shortest and easiest to use, consists of a three-day resting period and a three-day training period. The training period actually consists of two days of workouts followed by your competition day—which is also your scheduled peak.

Power lifter Jack Roybal of Alexandria, Virginia, put this cycle to the test when training for a power lifting meeting in Santa Fe, New Mexico, that was held July 9, 1988.

"I took off July 4, 5, and 6," he explains. "On the 7th I had a light workout, half the weight of my openers; on the 8th I went through the motions and did some stretching." On the 9th, the third day of gradually increasing his efforts, he won his weight class—in only the second competition he had ever entered.

Third-Day-Back Successes

If you search athletic records, you'll find numerous examples of athletes who have excelled following rest periods. On their third day back after their rest periods, they turned in great performances. All of the following people, although unaware of Consistent Winning, trained for periods that approximated the 3-Day Cycle after taking unplanned rest periods.

● World-class runner Allison Roe habitually takes Wednesdays off when racing on Saturdays, thus creating a *three-day* gradual increase to maximum performance.

● Brad Gilbert had lost to John McEnroe seven times. But on January 15, 1986, after being ill and unable to practice until *three days* before the match, Gilbert beat McEnroe in what sports reporters called the tennis match of Gilbert's life.

● *A few days before* Jesse Owens exploded one track and field world record after another at the Big Ten Championships in Ann Arbor, Michigan, on May 25, 1935, he'd been laid up with a sore back, unable to work out at all. Rather than "losing it" due to the inactivity, Owens tied the 100-yard dash record of 9.4 seconds, broke the long jump record and the 220-yard dash record, and set a record for the 220-yard hurdles.

● Remember Scott Morson from chapter 2? During his training for the Boston Marathon in 1980, Morson came down with a bad case of the flu and missed eight days of running. His first day back he ran 3 miles, the second day 4 miles. Then he panicked because the race was getting closer. The *third day back* he ran the fastest 20-mile training run he has ever done. It felt so easy he didn't realize how much faster than usual he was running, he says. Morson went on to run the Boston Marathon in 2:34.

● Deborah Jean Harding is a professional singer and musician. She says, "After I miss two or *three days* or more of singing, my first day of singing feels flat. The second day my voice is okay, and on the third day back, the timing of my voice and instrument is perfect."

● Lyn Brooks, at the time unaware of Consistent Winning, was tired the week before The Mighty Hamptons Triathlon (1.5-mile swim, 25-mile bike, 10-mile run) in September 1982. She had not trained much that week and missed a day of training *two days before the event*. The day before the event she ran 8 miles and biked 17, and she felt great. The next day she won the event.

How to Plan Your Peak

The 3-Day Cycle, with its three-day resting period followed by a three-day training period, must be scheduled five days before your event. For example, if you want to peak for a race June 30, you'd start the cycle June 25. Both of the longer cycles, the 3-Week and 3-Month Cycle, also end with a 3-Day Cycle.

The resting period consists of one day of active rest followed by two days of rest. This tapering-down period allows your body to be rested and readied for an all-out effort. Don't worry that your muscles will start to lose their conditioning. Studies have shown that muscle power increases every day during a week of gradually decreasing effort.

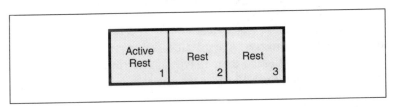

Three-Day Rest: *Remember that on an active rest day you can work out lightly for 30 minutes, while on rest days you can only go for walks.*

The training period begins with one day of easy training, followed by a day of easy to moderate training. The third day you go all out—this is your "peak" day, the day of your event. The two milder training days have provided what we call a "tapering-up" period to provide maximum performance on the third day of training.

To set up the 3-Day Cycle, count backward on your calendar, counting the day of the event (or first day of a long event) as "3," the day before the event as "2," and the day before that as "1." Day 1 is the first day of training in the 3-Day Cycle. Then count back another three days to lay out the resting period. If your event is on a Saturday, for instance, you begin training on Thursday.

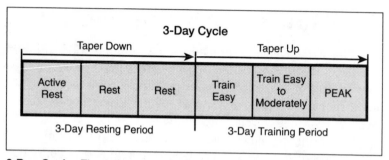

3-Day Cycle: *The 3-Day Cycle includes a three-day resting period and a three-day training period. You peak on the third day of resumed training.*

You Need Time to Taper

John Jerome, a long-time canoeist and raftsman and a contributing writer for *Outside* magazine, has noted that athletes are often more fit and reach their maximum performance one to two days after competition. Most likely this occurs because they have

SAMPLE 3-DAY CYCLE

For a marathon runner hoping to peak for an event on, say, October 22, a 3-Day Cycle—including resting and training periods—might look like this.

October 17: Active rest—20 to 30 minutes of easy running.

October 18: Rest—easy 30-minute walk or less.

October 19: Rest—easy 30-minute walk or less.

October 20: Training—½- to 1½-hour run, easy pace.

October 21: Training—1- to 1½-hour run, moderate pace.

October 22: Event day (your peak)—all out!

tapered down to a rest the day before the competition, which did not give their bodies sufficient time to work back up to peak performance levels. Resting the day before a competition does not allow your body enough time to get "revved" back up to a maximum efficiency. Instead, that day of rest literally sets up a peak period for two days *after* the event.

Although the 3-Day Cycle is designed to begin with a three-day resting period, it will work with much longer initial periods of rest—planned or not. It can even work with a one-day rest, although not as effectively. You might recall from your own experiences a time when you took a week or even ten days off with the flu or a mild injury. Had you been keeping records you likely would have found that on your third day back, you felt terrific.

CHAPTER EIGHT

THE 3-WEEK CYCLE: 21 DAYS TO PEAK PERFORMANCE

Even more dramatic results occur with the 3-Week Cycle of Consistent Winning. Nick Bassett used this cycle to train for the 1984 Western States 100-Mile, a tortuous run through the Rocky Mountains. Going into his third and fourth day of rest, he noted, "I began to feel so good physically that I realized for the first time how overtrained I really was." Bassett's 22-hour, 46-minute time not only was a personal best but also broke the record for Wyoming entrants.

Planned Performances

Other test athletes also found success with the 3-Week Cycle.

● Phil Kiner, world-class and five-time All-America trap-shooter, uses Consistent Winning by taking five resting days, then training *21 days* for his shooting matches. "I have more wins and a higher all-around average than ever," he says.

● Power lifter Jack Roybal used the *3-Week Cycle* to prepare for his first competition. He says, "As I kept improving toward my peak, the other fellows I worked out with all peaked early and kept dropping in performance as the event got closer." Roybal turned in a personal best performance and placed third. In the four years since, Roybal has continued to use the 3-Week and 3-Day Cycles, and has produced personal bests at *every competition* he has entered, all at the state or regional level.

• Dr. Peter Seitz, a veterinarian in Santa Fe, New Mexico, works out twice a day, usually seven days a week. He plays racquetball and rugby, runs, and lifts weights. He used the *3-Week Cycle* to prepare for a rugby tournament on April 22 and 23, 1988, in Austin, Texas. His taper-down and taper-up ended with 4 hours of sleep the night before the tournament, no supper, and lots of beer. Seitz said, "I played great all weekend. After the second game Saturday, I felt better than I usually do after one game. I played three games that day!"

• Rick Bishop is a highly trained marathon runner who was a member of the record-holding team for the Ultra Marathon Relay from Death Valley to Mount Whitney (from the lowest to the highest point in the continental United States) with a time of 38 hours, 35 minutes, 48 seconds. Looking forward to the 20-mile race of the 1984 Mayor's Cup Series in Denver, Colorado, he came down with the flu and missed his workouts 12 days in a row. Aware of the Consistent Winning technique, Bishop delayed beginning his training again after recovery for a day or two so that his event would fall on the *21st day back*. On day 21, after he resumed training, he won the race by a significant margin. His remark? "I don't know where it came from!"

• Lyn Brooks used the *3-Week Cycle* to capture her win in the 1984 Ultraman Triathlon, described at the beginning of this book. She peaked right on schedule, winning the double marathon and the event.

Accidental Peaks

Many athletes, unaware of Consistent Winning and its training and resting cycles, nonetheless peaked after "accidental" three-week training periods. The following athletes experienced such accidental peaks.

• After recovering from a torn ankle ligament, New Zealander Dick Taylor had only three weeks to train before the Commonwealth Games. At the end of his *third week* of workout, he won the 10,000-meter run.

• World-class runner Dave Bedford would sometimes train up to 200 or more miles a week. A hamstring injury, however, limited him to an average of 25 miles per week for three months in 1973. After *three weeks* of accelerated training, he then broke the world record for the 10,000-meter run.

• Tennis star Monica Seles, suffering from shin splints and a stress fracture, withdrew from Wimbledon on the eve of the 1991 championship. She did not play competitively for almost two months until the 1991 Pathmark Tennis Classic. Seles won her match 6-0, 6-2 and, according to newspaper reports, "proclaimed herself in great shape after *three weeks* of exercise and treatment."

Planning Ahead

The 3-Week Cycle begins with a five-day resting period and then is followed by exactly 21 days to a peak. Remember that October 22 race? To use the 3-Week Cycle, you'd begin your rest period September 27 and begin training October 2 to peak on October 22. The 21 days contain a 15-day training period and the 3-Day Cycle (three days of rest followed by three days of training) at the end. The 3-Week Cycle will work without the 3-Day Cycle at the end, but your performance will be even better if you include it.

To set up the 3-Week Cycle, count backward on your calendar, counting your event day as "21." The day before the event is "20" and so on back to day 1 to lay out the training period. Count back another five days to allow for the resting period. The entire cycle spans 26 days.

The initial five-day resting period consists of two rest days, one active rest day, then two more rest days. This five-day resting period must end 21 days before your desired peak. If absolutely necessary, you can lengthen or shorten the resting period, but

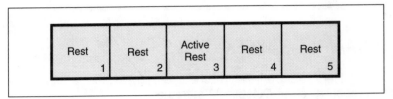

Five-Day Resting Period: _The 3-Week Cycle is kicked off with a five-day resting period._

remember that you must have two rest days before you start the training period.

To begin the cycle, take two days of rest. Follow that with one day of light activity, then two more days of rest. This constitutes the initial five-day resting period. You are now 21 days away from your peak.

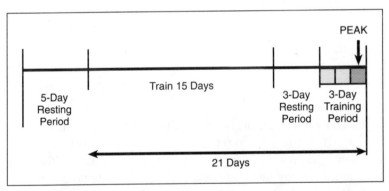

3-Week Cycle: _After the five-day rest, you train normally for 15 days, and then plug in a complete 3-Day Cycle, with resting and training periods. This cycle takes 21 days from beginning of training to peak performance._

After the rest period, always make sure your first two days back to training are very easy, even though you will almost certainly feel like going harder. If you hold back on those two days, you will have a stronger and higher peak on the third day, and reduce your chances of injury.

After resting, begin the training period by training for 15

SAMPLE 3-WEEK CYCLE

Here's how a training schedule might look for a runner preparing for an October 22 marathon.

September 27: Rest—easy 30-minute walk or less.
September 28: Rest—easy 30-minute walk or less.
September 29: Active rest—20 to 30 minutes of easy running.
September 30: Rest—Easy 30-minute walk or less.
October 1: Rest—Easy 30-minute walk or less.
October 2–16: 15 days of normal training (insert rest days if needed).
October 17: Active rest—20 to 30 minutes of easy running.
October 18: Rest—easy 30-minute walk or less.
October 19: Rest—easy 30-minute walk or less.
October 20: Training—½- to 1½-hour run, easy pace.
October 21: Training—1- to 1½-hour run, moderate pace.
October 22: Event day (your peak)—all out!

days. This doesn't mean, however, that you have to train 15 days straight. If you're used to training for 15 days in a row, fine, but you can insert rest days as needed. What's important is that you have the three-day resting period and three-day training period at the end of the cycle so you'll have an extra catapult effect for a peak performance on the last day.

After the 15 days your maximum performance day is still six days away, which allows enough time for the 3-Day Cycle. Plug in the 3-Day Cycle by tapering down with one day of active rest followed by two days of rest. Taper up again to a total of three days of activity. That third day, which is the end of both cycles, will be your maximum performance day, the day of your event. It will be the day you find yourself wondering, "Where did it come from?" as have other athletes who have used the Consistent Winning technique—whether they were aware of it or not.

CHAPTER NINE

THE 3-MONTH CYCLE: PLANNING FOR A MAJOR PEAK

The 3-Month Cycle, which includes *both* the 3-Week Cycle and 3-Day Cycle, will give you the strongest peak. Like the other cycles, it's kicked off with a rest period, but for this cycle the rest period is longer—13 days. Although 13 days sounds like an awfully long resting period, don't panic: It's actually two separate five-day rests with three days of training in between, and there is a total of five training days. As always, Consistent Winning never allots more than two rest days in a row—and remember that even those can include 30-minute walks. The longer resting periods of Consistent Winning always include training days.

Peaks in 12 Weeks

It's easy to find examples of athletes who regularly peak after 12-week or three-month training periods, and scientific studies confirm the efficacy of a 12-week training cycle. (Refer to "Maximal Improvement in 12 Weeks" on page 41.) Consider these examples:

• A study at the University of Jyvaskyla in Finland involved a test group of men doing squats three days a week for 16 weeks. The study revealed that electrical activity and muscle force in their quadriceps (the large thigh muscles) increased to a peak at *12 weeks,* and then decreased thereafter.

• Zola Budd Pieters, world-class runner, missed almost a year of training because of injuries. She returned to action in late September 1987, and won the Kodak Classic 10K in Northern Ireland in 32:17. After winning the race Pieters remarked to reporters, "I have been training for *three months* and feel much more relaxed."

• Bodybuilder Frank Zane, three-time Mr. Olympia, attributes his longevity to the use of two or three training cycles each year. He told *Muscle and Fitness* magazine: "Following the Mr. Olympia, I take a layoff and generally slow my training until the first of the year. Every January, I more or less start all over as a bodybuilder. I reach either two or three peaks every year, each peak higher than the last. I think that *three months* is a good period of time over which to reach a goal. Work through a three-month peaking phase, take a couple of days off training, then start another peaking cycle."

• Joan Benoit Samuelson is a great example of a true champion, a talented and hard-driven athlete. In late December 1981, she had Achilles tendon surgery. She had eight weeks away from running but kept in shape using a stationary bicycle and Nautilus equipment. She began running again, and by the late summer of 1982 (which amounted to two *3-Month Cycles* back-to-back), she produced an American record at 10 miles. At the Nike Marathon in Eugene, Oregon, she ran the fastest loop marathon in history.

Then because of knee problems and surgery, Samuelson had time off again for about a month, from mid-April to mid-May 1984, running only seven or eight days during those weeks. After training *12 weeks*, she won the Olympic marathon on August 5, 1984, cutting 47 seconds off the record.

Return to Training Cautiously

After peak times you should take a resting period or at least diminish your training to avoid illness, injury, or burnout. Track coach Nate Breen offers a good example of what can happen if you continue pushing past 12 weeks. After missing 48 days of running because of ankle surgery, Breen began training March 1, 1987. On April 5, just under five weeks later, he won the Boulder Memorial Hospital Run. In the 12th week of training, he made this note in his diary: "All runs super, blasting through the park."

After 12½ weeks, still pushing, he tore his calf muscle at the Bolder Boulder Race in Colorado. A resting period after three months of training, as outlined in the Consistent Winning technique, would have averted this injury. Breen heartily agrees.

After a resting period or after you have missed training for any reason, it's important to come back slowly. Most people who have had a few weeks or more off for any reason are cautious when returning to their sport, because the chances for injury are increased after layoffs. It is important that the first few days back to training are very easy, building gradually to harder workouts.

If you miss two weeks of training, allow yourself two weeks to gradually get back to your former level. The third week will be at a higher level of performance than when you ended your workouts.

Laying the Foundation

If you want to really peak at the end of 12 weeks, you must allow your body to detrain sufficiently before you begin your buildup. If not, you will lose the gift of biochemical peaking that comes naturally with this timing. After an extended rest, resumed training will bring your body's aerobic physiology to true peak performance levels in 12 weeks.

The extended rest necessary to set up the three-month training period is called the 13-day resting period, but it is actually two separate five-day resting periods with three days of training in between. There are a total of five days of action mixed in with eight days of rest, which means you never have more than two rest days in a row.

The 13-day resting period begins with two rest days, followed by an active rest day and two more rest days. Then come three training days, followed by two rest days, an active rest day, and two more rest days. Remember that an active rest day may include a 20- to 30-minute light workout, while a regular rest day should have no workout more strenuous than a 30-minute walk.

One way to think of the 13-day resting period is to compare it to planting a seed. After planting, you go about your business and eventually find that the seed springs up, grows, and, in time, bears its fruit.

Note that three training days are included in the middle of the rest period. The 3-Month Cycle is the only one where regular training days break up a resting period.

Marking It Off

The 3-Month Cycle is actually a cycle sandwich: An extended training period of 34 days, or five weeks, is flanked on either side

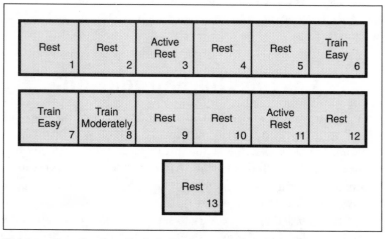

Thirteen-Day Resting Period: *Don't worry! You don't rest the entire 13 days. There are three training days and two active rest days scheduled.*

by 3-Week Cycles. In the final 3-Week Cycle, t.
form a 3-Day Cycle.

Incorporating the 3-Month Cycle means starting y
period 84 days before the event and starting the resting ,   .3
days before that. So you'll need 97 days, or a bit more than three
months, for this cycle. Find the day of the event on your calendar,
mark it as "84," the day before the event as "83," and so on
until you've reached 1. Now count back 13 more days to mark
off your 13-day resting period.

Once past the 13-day rest, actively train for 21 days. Again,
if you don't normally train this many days in a row, don't hesitate
to add rest days when needed.

Then take a three-day resting period (one day of active rest
and two rest days). Next, actively train for 34 days, again inserting
rest days if your body demands them. But be aware that training
more than about five weeks can have negative consequences: It
will reduce rather than enhance your performance. So take another
five-day resting period to set up the final 3-Week Cycle. Finally,
fill in the three days of resting followed by three days of training
that make up the final 3-Day Cycle.

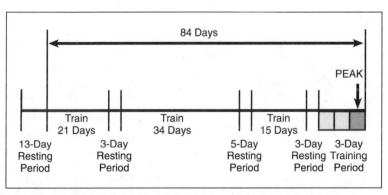

3-Month Cycle: *The 3-Month Cycle incorporates both the 3-Week Cycle and the 3-Day Cycle. This cycle starts off with the 13-day resting period, so you need 97 days from start to peak.*

TRAINING FOR THE BIG ONE

Aiming at a big event in October, and it's midsummer now? You start off July 18 with the 13-day resting period (remember that there are several light training days within this long resting period). This cycle features training periods of 21 days, 34 days, 15 days, and 3 days, but you can add extra rest days within these training periods if needed.

July

S	M	T	W	T	F	S
					1	2
3	4	5	6	7	8	9
10	11	12	13	14	15	16
17	18 Rest	19 Rest	20 Active Rest	21 Rest	22 Rest	23 Train Easy
24 Train Easy	25 Train Moderately	26 Rest	27 Rest	28 Active Rest	29 Rest	30 Rest
31						

August

S	M	T	W	T	F	S
	1	2	3	4	5	6
7	8	9	10	11	12	13
14	15	16	17	18	19	20
21 Active Rest	22 Rest	23 Rest	24	25	26	27
28	29	30	31			

September

S	M	T	W	T	F	
				1 🏃	2 🏃	🏃
4 🏃	5 🏃	6 🏃	7 🏃	8 🏃	9 🏃	10 🏃
11 🏃	12 🏃	13 🏃	14 🏃	15 🏃	16 🏃	17 🏃
18 🏃	19 🏃	20 🏃	21 🏃	22 🏃	23 🏃	24 🏃
25 🏃	26 🏃	27 Rest	28 Rest	29 Active Rest	30 Rest	

October

S	M	T	W	T	F	S
						1 Rest
2 🏃	3 🏃	4 🏃	5 🏃	6 🏃	7 🏃	8 🏃
9 🏃	10 🏃	11 🏃	12 🏃	13 🏃	14 🏃	15 🏃
16 🏃	17 Active Rest	18 Rest	19 Rest	20 Train Easy	21 Train Easy	22 PEAK
23	24	25	26	27	28	29
30	31					

🏃 = Training Day

CHAPTER TEN

PUSHING TOO LONG DOESN'T PAY

You will note that at no time does Consistent Winning advocate training past five weeks without taking a resting period. You cannot train effectively at the same level more than five weeks without a resting period. If you do so, performance decreases, and chances for injuries increase. Using the five-week mark as the time for a "corrective" wave to begin a new cycle occurs in many aspects of life other than sports.

This is true for followers of artistic disciplines as well. Jim Rabby of Santa Fe, New Mexico, is a prolific fine artist. His canvases hang in the collections of hundreds of major corporations as well as in private galleries and homes. He has painted action scenes of Joe Namath, Rod Laver, Gordie Howe, and Billie Jean King and a portrait of Hank Aaron after his 715th home run. He has painted collections for former president Lyndon Johnson and the Smithsonian Air and Space Museum. Rabby says he sometimes paints as much as 14 hours a day, every day. But he says, "After five or six weeks, I must take time off. It feels as though I can't focus. I have a lack of direction. I'm not true to my inner clock."

Most people are not as "tuned" to their inner clock as Rabby; they have to rely on the calendar to let them know when it is time for a rest. But that does not mean that the inner clock isn't ticking—it is, whether you are aware of it or not.

You Can Only Push for So Long

Another example of this five-week maximum is Sebastian Coe's unexpected defeat in an 800-meter race in September 1982. Coe, the world record holder in the 800, had looked good in all three of his races since coming back from a leg injury the previous month, and had cruised to easy victories in his earlier heats. Injuries, however, had fragmented his training schedule that year. Coe told reporters, "I always knew that after only five weeks of training, sooner or later the body would break."

Coe's defeat occurred immediately beyond the five weeks of training and racing. He started training too early and peaked too soon. Proper timing of resting and training periods as laid out in Consistent Winning would have helped prevent this misfortune.

You can find numerous other occurences of this "peak-too-soon" phenomena, both in athletes and in exercise physiology labs, such as the following examples.

● Although Nick Bassett had used the 3-Week Cycle to achieve his personal best in the 1984 Western States 100-Mile Run, he felt so strong while training for the same event in 1985 that he opted to train through to the end, taking no rest at all. He had five hard weekends of racing before the 100-miler, achieving great performances, including several personal bests. But after *five weeks* without a resting period, his performance declined. He barely finished the race in 25 hours and 30 minutes, almost 3 hours longer than he had taken the year before. "Thirty minutes into the race, I knew I didn't have it," Bassett says.

● Kevin A. Mikesell and Gary Dudley at the Chicago College of Osteopathic Medicine and Ohio University in Athens did a study of the effect of intense endurance training on the aerobic power of well-conditioned competitive distance runners. They measured the runners' aerobic power and found that it increased during the first five weeks. Aerobic power *decreased after five weeks* and decreased significantly after week 6.

• Nancy Broun Bates of Houston, Texas, an aerobics instructor, had regularly taught and exercised six days a week for 12 years. To all of this activity she suddenly added a weekly Level 3 aerobic bench class, an intense workout that calls for stepping up and down on a 12-inch platform while doing various routines. Bates says, "I felt great after the additional class until after *five weeks*. All of a sudden I hurt badly afterward. I felt like I had the flu. I ached badly all over and felt sick but knew I didn't have the flu. It would last a couple of days, then I was fine. After three weeks of feeling bad each time, I skipped the class, recovered, and felt great."

Don't be fooled by how good you feel: "Pushing through" beyond five straight weeks of training always takes its toll, usually when you can afford it least. If you are training too hard it may not even take five weeks to notice your decreased level of performance. Remember Steve in chapter 2? He suddenly increased his daily running mileage by over one-third and broke down physically after three weeks of his new regimen.

Rather than work against the natural cycles of nature, take a rest after five weeks, as you follow the three-five-three week pattern. Your body will regroup its forces and catapult you forward to consistently high performances.

Training Less for Better Results

There is more to taking a resting period than setting up the timing cycles. As Clarence Bass, international physique judge, writer, and bodybuilding competitor, states in his book *Ripped 2,* "The less I train, the better I become." Although it may be difficult to accept this as reality, it has been proven time and again that *once your training base is established, timing of when to rest becomes the more important element.*

Exercise physiologist David Costill, Ph.D., has discovered that there is a limit beyond which athletes cease to improve. After measuring the performance of beginning, average, and elite athletes at Ball State University in Muncie, Indiana, Dr. Costill concluded the optimal maximum training mileage for runners is

50 to 75 weekly miles. Beyond that, the amount of physiological improvement was virtually insignificant, he says, even at 225 miles per week, and endurance was not improved. Other athletes, such as the following, have also found that training less for better results pays off.

• John Treacy of Ireland won the silver medal for the marathon at the 1984 Olympics in 2:09:56. His long training run each week was 20 miles, at a relatively slow 8-minute pace.

• After long-time runner, writer, and cardiologist George Sheehan, M.D., shifted from six days of running per week to three days, he ran his best marathon—at age 62.

• Young bowler Henry Sandoval, 15, had been practicing bowling six days a week, ten games a day—until he dislocated his thumb. He hadn't bowled in months when he went to the 1987 YABA Junior State Bowling Tournament in New Mexico, where he rolled a perfect 300 game. Sandoval said that taking time off bowling helped immensely, telling reporters, "Everything I did was right."

CHAPTER ELEVEN

ADVANCED SCHEDULING

In some cases, you may want to plan farther ahead than the 3-Month Cycle, or you may find that your competition schedule won't fit neatly into the Consistent Winning cycles discussed so far. Because of the complexity of competition schedules, you can't always use the basic cycles. They can be adapted, however, to fit most schedules. In the following pages you'll find specific instructions on how to do so.

Multiple-Day Events

If you have a multiple-day event such as the Ultraman Triathlon, which runs three days in a row, schedule the first day of the event as your maximum performance day. This applies to whichever cycle you use. High performance can be maintained for up to two weeks beyond the 3-Week Cycle.

With special preparation, you can maintain high performance for an entire month. This kind of high performance maintenance is useful for long events such as the Olympics, the Olympic trials, or the Tour de France bicycle race.

To set up for a monthlong event, make a schedule with eight

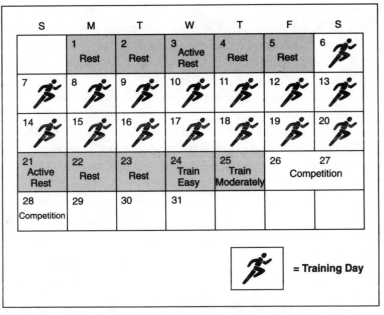

	S	M	T	W	T	F	S
		1 Rest	2 Rest	3 Active Rest	4 Rest	5 Rest	6
	7	8	9	10	11	12	13
	14	15	16	17	18	19	20
	21 Active Rest	22 Rest	23 Rest	24 Train Easy	25 Train Moderately	26 Competition	27
	28 Competition	29	30	31			

= Training Day

Multiple-Day Events: *To compete in events that run several days, you start with a five-day resting period, train 15 days, rest for three, and then you're into the final three-day training period. The last day of that period is your peak—and the first day of your event.*

training days leading up to your event. Before that eight-day training period, plug in a five-day resting period (two days off, one on, two off). The eighth training day is the first day of your event and is a high-performance day. You then have four more weeks during which you can race and stay at high performance.

Planning for a Major Event

When preparing for a major event, you should plan far enough ahead so you can group two 3-Month Cycles. A double 3-Month Cycle stacks two 3-Month Cycles back-to-back and is the best timing procedure to use for a major event. You must have enough time, however, for both 3-Month Cycles plus the 13-day resting period before the first cycle, and if possible, another 13-day rest between cycles. Thirteen days is optimal for the rest period, but five days is the *minimum* effective resting period. Back-to-back 3-Month Cycles, in effect, must be planned over half a year before a given event.

If you were planning for an event in the fall—such as the Ironman on October 22—you would need to start with a 13-day resting period April 12, and would begin training April 25. (Refer to "Training for the Big One" on page 66 to see how a 3-Month Cycle is set up.) You'd have a major peak July 17, and then would take another 13-day resting period before starting your second 3-Month Cycle July 31 for an October 22 peak. (You would also have several minor peaks: on April 27, May 15 and 21, June 8 and 29, August 2, 20, and 26, September 13, and October 4.)

Triple 3-Month Cycles

The performances of Frank Zane, three-time Mr. Olympia, coincide with the Consistent Winning triple cycle. He reaches either two or three peaks every year, each peak higher than the last. He works through a three-month peaking phase, takes a few days off training, then starts another peaking cycle.

The triple 3-Month Cycle is perfect for planning for an upcoming season. Train to build a base during the first 3-Month Cycle—this means train steadily, but don't go all out. During the second 3-Month Cycle, add intensity to increased training. The third 3-Month Cycle is your competitive season. To count off triple cycles, count your target peak performance day as "84," the day before it as "83," and so on. (See "Marking It Off" on page 64.) Repeat this counting-off process three times, until you have all three 3-Month Cycles marked off.

After a triple 3-Month Cycle, take a few months for recovery and easy training so that you can begin another triple 3-Month Cycle with a good rest base. You need a minimum of six easy weeks to allow your body time to recover.

If injury, surgery, or illness causes you to lose three or more

months of activity, use triple 3-Month Cy
periods in between to bring yourself back t
formance. Triple 3-Month Cycles create pro
peaks for an explosion of power at the end; how
beyond a triple cycle without significant rest will decre
mance and increase chances for injury.

Holding a Peak

There may be times when you want to participate in competitions on consecutive weekends. If your competition days are
Saturdays, you would set up the appropriate resting and training
cycle to peak on the first event day of the season. The day after
your competition—in this case Sunday—would be a rest day.

You would then train easy on Monday and hard on Tuesday.
Wednesday would be a rest day to set up a modified 3-Day Cycle
(with only one rest day instead of two). Train easy on Thursday

	S	M	T	W	T	F	S
Week 1	Rest	🏃	🏃	Rest	🏃	🏃	Compete
Week 2	Rest	🏃	🏃	Rest	🏃	🏃	Compete
Week 3	Rest	🏃	🏃	Rest	🏃	🏃	Compete
Week 4	Rest	Active Rest or Train Easy	Rest	Rest	🏃	🏃	Compete
Week 5	Rest	🏃	🏃	Rest	🏃	🏃	Compete

🏃 = Training Day

Peaking Consecutive Weekends: *To peak every weekend for five weeks, you'd rest two days a week. After three weeks, however, you'd need to insert two extra rest days to avoid overuse problems.*

PEAKING FOR A WHOLE SEASON

To continue to peak each weekend for an entire three-month season, you'd add additional rest days during week 4, week 9, and week 13. These extra rest days lessen the chances of injuries as well as ensure that the cycles work.

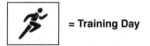 = Training Day

	S	M	T	W	T	F	S
Week 1	Compete	Rest	Train	Train	Rest	Train	Train
Week 2	Compete	Rest	Train	Train	Rest	Train	Train
Week 3	Compete	Rest	Train	Train	Rest	Train	Train
Week 4	Compete	Rest	Active Rest or Train Easy	Rest	Rest	Train	Train
Week 5	Compete	Rest	Train	Train	Rest	Train	Train

and with increasing intensity on Friday. Saturday is competition day and should yield another peak performance.

You can follow this schedule for three weeks in a row. At that point, in the fourth week, take Tuesday off to lengthen the resting period. Monday can be an active rest day if your competition wasn't too intense.

This translates to a simple formula: Rest Sundays and Wednesdays to compete on consecutive Saturdays. (If your com-

	S	M	T	W	T	F	S
Week 6	Compete	Rest	Train	Train	Rest	Train	Train
Week 7	Compete	Rest	Train	Train	Rest	Train	Train
Week 8	Compete	Rest	Train	Train	Rest	Train	Train
Week 9	Compete	Rest	Active Rest or Train Easy	Rest	Rest	Train	Train
Week 10	Compete	Rest	Train	Train	Rest	Train	Train

	S	M	T	W	T	F	S
Week 11	Compete	Rest	Train	Train	Rest	Train	Train
Week 12	Compete	Rest	Train	Train	Rest	Train	Train
Week 13	Compete	Rest	Active Rest or Train Easy	Rest	Rest	Train	Train
Week 14	Compete	Rest	Train	Train	Rest	Train	Train
Week 15	Compete	Rest	Train	Train	Rest	Train	Train

petition days are Sundays, you can alter the schedule so you rest Mondays and Thursdays.) Each week there are two rest days and five training days, including the competition day.

The rest day after intense competition is crucial. You must rest after stress to recover for the next workout. In an extreme example, researchers at the Human Performance Laboratory at Ball State University in Muncie, Indiana, and the Work Physiology Laboratory at Ohio State University in Columbus examined

...ed male runners for one week after the
...l records in a marathon. The runners who
...no running during the previous week re-
...nd work capacity more rapidly than those
...45 minutes daily during that week.

Peaking Every Week

This repetitive scheduling can also be used for professional football players or other pro athletes. Because the games are on Sunday, these athletes would rest Mondays and Thursdays to set up a 3-Day Cycle for a peak the following Sunday.

During the fourth week of the season, add Tuesday and Wednesday as rest days. Then continue with the Monday and Thursday resting formula.

Research, as mentioned in chapter 10, has proven that you

HIGH- AND LOW-PERFORMANCE DAYS

Throughout any training period, you can expect highs and lows on certain days. Knowing when to expect the peak days will help you schedule your training program.

High-performance days consistently occur after any resting period on the third day back to training (3-Day Cycle), the 21st day (3-Week Cycle), the end of the fifth week, and the end of the 12th week of training (3-Month Cycle).

Certain other days after resting tend to be high performance—the fifth day, eighth day, and the whole third week after a rest. Some days seem sluggish, although the sluggish days are not as definite or as reliably predictable as peak days. The exception is if you are overtraining. There is a good chance you will get sick or develop an overuse injury after three weeks or after five weeks from when you started overdoing it.

cannot train heavily beyond five weeks and retain high performance. You need to add a four-day resting period, which includes some active rest, during week 9 of the season, extending from Monday to Thursday. This particular timing allows the necessary detraining and provides a 3-Day Cycle that ends with a peak performance on Sunday.

This four-day resting period shown in the fourth week is first taken after the initial three weeks. The resting period is repeated after four more weeks of training and competing, then three weeks, then four, and so forth. This scheduling will keep performance high and keep you peaking on time, help avoid injury and illness, and prevent an overtraining effect.

Remember, most weeks you are training or competing five days a week. Take a resting period after the first three weeks of your season, then alternate the four-day rests every three and four weeks. If you're overextended physically, take the four-day resting period every three weeks.

For athletes who normally work out twice a day, seven days a week and are hesitant to add rest days, remember the example of Dave Scott's Ironman victories mentioned in chapter 1. Scott set a course record in 1986 following many periods of three to five days off, and won again in 1987, following more periods of days off.

CHAPTER TWELVE

PREPARING TO WIN

The cycles of Consistent Winning are designed to produce peak performances when desired and to lessen the chances of injury, illness, and burnout from overextending yourself. To maximize your chances for top performances and to minimize the chances for injury, it's imperative that you regularly warm up for your workouts as well as your races, and cool down afterward.

Getting Ready

Warming up is a transition period from inactivity to activity, and this transition follows the same natural up-and-down cyclic patterns as other human performance. Failure to properly warm up increases chances for injury. Cold muscles can cramp and tear, and tendons can rupture from quick, powerful movements when not properly warmed up.

A thorough warm-up not only can help prevent injuries but also can improve performances. As far back as 1947, researchers found a better response to a 15-minute warm-up than to a 5-minute warm-up. They found that a 15- to 30-minute warm-up yielded a 3 to 6 percent improvement in performance over all distances from the 100-meter dash to the 800-meter race.

Research reported in *Medicine and Science in Sports and Exercise* demonstrated that stretching for 20 minutes before a race yielded performance times that were 3 to 5 percent faster than without stretching. The longer the race distance, the higher the percentage of improvement. Stretching helps efficiency in any performance that requires muscular effort.

You should warm up by alternating your activity with stretching. Runners alternate running and stretching; dancers alternate dancing and stretching. The following example of warming up for a running race can be adapted to warming up for any muscular activity.

Begin to warm your body with an easy run, slowly working up to a moderate level. Then stretch to decrease activity, and finally run again to increase activity to a warm-up high. It is important to remember that you must begin with a slow warm-up to have a fast race.

For an effective warm-up that lasts about 30 minutes, begin with an easy 13-minute run. This warms the body and allows better and safer stretching. Next, stretch for 13 to 21 minutes. This stretching period creates a "valley" of rest, yet maintains circulation and warmth for flexibility. The final buildup to the warm-up high is a 5-minute run. After the final 5-minute run, your body is ready to perform more efficiently. You should finish your warm-up at the starting line as close to the start of the race as possible.

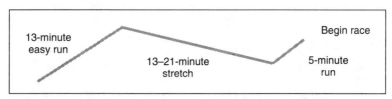

Warm-Up for a Running Race: *An effective warm-up for any physical activity follows natural cyclic patterns. For a running race, this would include an easy buildup, stretching, and another buildup to a warm-up peak.*

HOW TO LISTEN TO YOUR BODY

All of us have experienced days when we feel lazy and just don't want to work out. You may think that you ought to work out, but your body seems to be saying no. What should you do?

Try an easy warm-up for at least 13 minutes. It's possible that you'll feel below par at first, but after about 13 minutes things will begin to click, and you'll start feeling fine. You've probably had this happen before: You start off feeling sluggish and then have a terrific workout once you're into it.

It happens to people at every level of performance. Pitching ace Nolan Ryan felt miserable the evening he had his first no-hitter, back in 1973. In pregame warm-up his performance was so bad he told the bullpen pitchers to start warming up. To say that Ryan clicked after his warm-up is an understatement.

He did it again on May 1, 1991, when at age 44 he threw his seventh no-hitter. Before that game he told his pitching coach, "I feel old today. My back, head, heel, and middle finger hurt. I don't feel good." Ryan proceeded to strike out 16 batters and shut down the Toronto Blue Jays, at the time the best-hitting team in the major leagues. After the game he told reporters, "I had the best command of all three pitches. This is my most overpowering night."

Many people experience this phenomenon. Despite a headache, chills, and fever, Milwaukee Brewers pitcher Ted Higuera held the Kansas City Royals hitless September 1, 1987, before allowing one hit in the eighth inning.

As long as you're healthy, the easy 13-minute warm-up will tell you whether or not to continue or just have an easy workout. If after about 13 minutes you still feel miserable, then slow down or quit. On the days that you "don't have it" in training, there is no need to do your regular routine. Do what you can without taxing yourself. This is where your body is trying to tell you something. You are better off slowing down, knowing that the next day you will feel better. When you sense that something is wrong, don't push yourself or don't work out.

Occasionally, this phenomenon will work the other way. You feel good during the warm-up but never get in the groove during training. This is normal. Not all days in a training period are great performance days.

Why It Works

Warming up helps your body switch fuels—from using mostly muscle glycogen to using mostly fatty acids. This is what you need for events that demand endurance, such as events that last over 2 hours.

During the early part of an exercise period, the muscles draw mostly on glycogen, a chemical that is stored inside the muscle cells and converted to glucose (simple sugar) for fuel. Later in the exercise period, the muscles rely mostly on liver glycogen and fatty acids from fat cells for energy. Some protein in the liver is also used as an energy source. During long endurance exercise, more glucose is made in the liver from sources other than glycogen, such as lactate, glycerol, and protein.

Between 5 and 15 percent of the energy sources that sustain long endurance exercise come from protein. Proteins are made of amino acids, and there are 16 amino acids in the liver that can be converted into glucose. The contribution of protein as an energy source increases during long endurance events. The actual amount of protein used depends on the level of aerobic training of the individual and the intensity and duration of the exercise. A proper warm-up gets these efficient systems of energy production into action.

Improving Flexibility

Stretching is also important for preventing soft tissue injury and improving performance. Soft tissue includes the muscles, tendons, ligaments, cartilage, and other related connective tissues, such as the membranes surrounding the bones.

Connective tissue contains live cells that secrete flexible proteins called collagen and elastin. These proteins are laid down along the lines of force that occur when the connective tissue is stretched. This tissue needs to be supple and responsive to the forces exerted on it during physical activity.

Stretching also opens small blood vessels that nourish the connective tissue. Along with nearby muscular movement, this increases the temperature of the tissue. Increased body heat changes the molecular conformation of collagen and elastin, making them more springy and resilient. Warming up and stretching help prevent connective tissue tears that could result from quick, forceful movements during exercise. Such tears are more likely to occur when the tissue is cold.

Stretching without Harm

Safe stretching includes avoiding the stimulation of the stretch reflex. This reflex is triggered when a muscle is quickly stretched, as when you bounce. The muscle reacts by forcefully contracting and will not allow an effective stretch. This contracting reflex is a safety mechanism, built into the muscles and nervous system to keep the muscles from getting injured by sudden, quick, bouncy movements before they are warmed up and ready. To avoid the stretch reflex, use gentle, gradual static stretches.

Gentle, static stretches develop good flexibility. Hold a stretched position just short of discomfort for 13 to 21 seconds. Focus on your breathing: Breathe in deeply through the nose before you start holding the stretch, and then slowly expel air out through your mouth as you hold. As you are stretching, relax and allow your muscles to slowly lose their tension.

When your tension has subsided, stretch just a bit further to increase or develop your flexible range of motion. This is called a developmental stretch. Stay just under the point of pain: Hold the stretch another 13 to 21 seconds. Stretching to improve flexibility is best done just after aerobic exercise.

Warming up adequately allows you to stretch harder to develop greater flexibility, with less chance of injury. Areas of your body that should be stretched include your upper body, lower back, abdomen, quadriceps, hamstrings, and calves.

Finishing Up

Cooling down is a transition from strenuous activity to a slower state. Take a few minutes to slowly jog, bike, or swim—

MATCH YOUR EFFORTS TO YOUR NATURAL RHYTHM

Allowing for natural patterns can be a powerful addition to your race strategy. For example, in a marathon run, the first 2 miles of the race should be run well below a planned average pace. Running a race slowly at first and gradually increasing the pace fits with natural patterns of human performance. For longer races you must always start slower and run faster later for best results. For shorter races, however, you should be thoroughly warmed up and virtually at race pace from the start.

There is a good reason for warming up carefully and for starting slowly in long races and gradually increasing the workload. During the first few minutes of running, your body functions anaerobically—producing energy without using oxygen. Then aerobic systems begin to kick in, using oxygen to burn body fuel to make energy available to your muscles. After a few minutes of gradually increasing activity, the emphasis shifts from anaerobic to aerobic metabolism. A good warm-up begins this process, so by the time you begin your race you're already shifting to aerobic metabolism.

Miruts Yifter, a world-class runner, has won two Olympic and four World Cup gold medals by starting a race running relatively slowly and then finishing fast. Learn to pace yourself properly in a race. Don't get caught in the "bum's rush" at the starting gun by going out too fast. Concentrate on what you need to do—running your own preplanned pacing.

or whatever your activity is—after a strenuous or long effort. Cooling down is important for a number of physiological reasons.

During exercise, blood vessels expand in order to supply the working muscles with a rich blood supply. The blood supply, of course, carries oxygen and nutrients to the muscles, while carting off waste products of metabolism such as carbon dioxide and lactic acid. During exercise, there is also an increase in nerve stimulation and a surge of stress hormones, such as adrenaline and corticosteroids. This nerve stimulation and the stress hormones are needed to mobilize glucose and other fuel, such as fatty acids, for the working muscles to function at high levels of energy output. The increased nerve stimulation and stress hormones help to dilate the peripheral blood vessels as well.

If you abruptly stop moving after high-intensity exercise, your nerve stimulation and stress hormones are at a level too high for the decreased activity. Since one of the functions of hormones is dilating the blood vessels, the result is pooling of blood in the legs and swollen limbs. Pooling of blood, known as hemostasis, slows down the circulation or return of blood from the limbs to the heart and lungs.

Hemostasis slows the delivery of oxygen and nutrients to the recently worked muscles and inhibits the clearing of waste products. For example, carbon dioxide is not transported to the lungs for exhalation as quickly as if the legs were kept moving during a cool-down run. The delay in clearing the waste products of metabolism along with the stress hormone residue contributes to peripheral swelling, or edema. Edema is often painful and an indication that something is wrong with the body or the way the body is getting rid of fluid.

Hemostasis and edema are easy to avoid by taking the time to cool down. Cooling down is a vital part of winding down your high-intensity exercise session. It may take 5 to 13 minutes or more, depending on the duration and intensity of your exercise and your level of fitness. The longer and more intense your exercise, the longer it takes to cool down. However, the more fit you are, the faster you will return to a resting state.

CHAPTER THIRTEEN

MORE WINNING TECHNIQUES

Consistent Winning, of course, doesn't guarantee success all on its own. It's important to pay attention to all aspects of your training—including such important adjuncts as diet, mental techniques, and other training. Two training aids that may prove particularly useful are specificity of training—specific training aimed at improving one or two aspects of your sport—and cross training.

Specific Training

Specificity of training is aimed at developing certain specialized skills. It is training that focuses on specific body motions and body systems, making them stronger, more efficient, and/or more accurate than they would otherwise become from regular training or practice. Specific training divides the total action of your sport into parts. The focused training of those individual parts makes the total action easier, and helps you reach your goal more quickly. It works like Henry Ford's idea for building cars faster and more efficiently: Separate a large job into small parts and work on them individually. For example, by adding specificity of training to your running, you can fine-tune your training for a smoother and faster stride. A tennis player can develop a stronger and more accurate tennis stroke, or a dancer can develop a more perfect step than from regular routine practice.

Suppose you're a marathon runner who has logged many training miles and has great endurance, but you're not happy with your speed. Sprint workouts will increase speed. (You'll find examples of detailed specific workouts in chapter 14.) A tennis player can use weights or wall pulleys to develop more strength for a specific stroke. A football quarterback throwing a football through a tire swinging from a tree sharpens his ability to hit a receiver.

Training can be so specific that some motor skills obtained from training in one sport may not help you very much in another sport. On the other hand, cardiovascular and strength aspects of training are more generous and allow crossover benefits.

Training causes the neuromotor systems of your body to learn to do exactly what they practice doing. Very little of the specific motor skill developed in one sport will transfer to another sport. This phenomenon can be demonstrated when an experienced bicycle rider, with no running experience, goes for a run. Despite his high degree of training, he would get out of breath more quickly than would be expected for someone at his fitness level. This may be due to activation of a different pattern of mechanical sensors in his muscles that stimulate breathing rate. If you run 5 miles a day at an 8-minute-per-mile pace and rarely alter your training, you'll get good at running 5 miles a day at an 8-minute-per-mile pace. An attempt to run that same distance a minute per mile faster would prove difficult because your body hasn't experienced a 7-minute pace. If you're preparing for a marathon, you need to run at your planned marathon pace one or two times a week. (See "Your Marathon Pace" on page 94.)

There is a crossover in the development of a more efficient oxygen uptake system and stronger muscles. This benefit is realized by cross training between bicycling and running. Bicycling can help develop and maintain a runner's cardiovascular system while reducing the pounding that frequent long runs entail.

HOW SPECIFIC TRAINING HELPED ONE RUNNER

Marathon runner John Dietrich trained an average of 10 miles a day from 1978 to 1982, usually at the same pace, with five years in a row of 3,650 miles a year. His only speedwork was at races. Here's his account of adding specific training and the Consistent Winning technique to his workouts.

"Mixing in speedwork has helped me get back some of the speed I used to have in my younger years—not only helping get back lost speed but helping me get into shape for racing quicker. One advantage I feel with adding speedwork is that it helps my running form, makes me feel like I'm running smoother in races, and makes the race feel easier. It helps me especially if I do it right up to the race.

"Taking days off before a buildup to a race helps to peak for specific races. I feel mended and recovered. Hitting the peak day on race day as I have done several times in the past few years is exciting. You run a good race to a great race and, with the speedwork mixed in, actually have a kick at the end. That's a good feeling to have at the end of a race.

"The days off also help with the mental rest as well. It helps relieve the mental pressure of going out and pounding out another workout—_a truly total rest of mind and body on days off._"

Cumulative Effect

Specific workouts can be individually targeted toward development of strength, flexibility, aerobic capacity, speed, and endurance. By working on them individually, you can put everything together to produce a stronger performance on a competition day than you did in any one training workout. You're building a cumulative effect so you can excel on race days. For example, most runners are aware that just from routine same-speed and same-distance running they can sometimes triple the distance of their average run with no problem because of the cumulative effect of their training runs. (This effect is known as the Collapse Point Theory.)

By individually building up strength, speed, and endurance in separate specific workouts, you can put them all together for a superior racing performance.

Specific training, however, is not for the beginner in many cases. A runner needs a seven- or eight-month training base of at least 15 to 20 miles a week before attempting some of the specific workouts. Specific training should be worked into gradually—too much, too soon increases your chances for illness and injury.

How Does It Work?

With specific training, the particular body systems, tissues, and organs that you use in performing increase their capacity in the direction of your training. At your present level of conditioning, your muscles perform at the workload they are trained for and in the manner they are trained for. At this level your body is able to process a certain amount of fuel and oxygen (aerobic capacity) and deliver a certain amount of speed with a certain amount of efficiency. Nerve to muscle patterns (neuromotor pathways) have been trained to move your body with a certain level of speed and accuracy. Specifically performing the motions of your sport helps you develop both smoothness and precision. This fine-tunes the neuromotor pathways from the brain to the body parts involved in the motions. A musician may practice the same bar of music over and over, then practice another—and finally put them all together.

Body efficiency and accuracy become very specific with the training you're doing. Specific training allows you to increase each one of these system's capacities individually toward the way you want to use them—without going all out in training as you would in competition. If you don't overtrain, you'll be able to recover quicker and have another quality workout the next day.

Specific training takes these systems and muscles of your

body above and beyond (or at least equal to) the demands you encounter in competition. So when you put all of your training together on competition day, your body *is familiar with and has adapted to* the stresses from the high performance you are demanding.

Mixing Consistent Winning with Cross Training

You can also benefit from cross training, training in two or more activities. Many athletes use cross training because it keeps them fit while partially resting and balancing certain muscles that are used more in one of their sports than the other. The Consistent Winning technique can be used with cross training as well as training for just one sport—it works regardless of the number of sports or activities you participate in. It works if you're training for the three events of a triathlon, or alternating days of weight training with trapshooting as Phil Kiner does, or combining racquetball, running, weight training, and rugby as Peter Seitz does.

During the second of three games of a rugby tournament in Aspen, Colorado, Seitz had to take a break. After a brief rest and some food, however, he was revitalized, and a great game followed. "I have never recovered like that before after feeling down," said Seitz. He had prepared with the 3-Week and 3-Day Cycles and with his four-sport cross training.

In summary, cross training can help you avoid becoming stale or overworking certain muscle groups, while specificity of training refines certain motions or techniques. Either or both of them, used in conjunction with Consistent Winning, will help you to attain superb performances.

CHAPTER FOURTEEN

JUST FOR RUNNERS

To give an example of detailed, specific training, we've developed some recommendations for runners.

In this chapter, we recommend three basic runs: the anaerobic threshold run, sprints, and the carbohydrate depletion run. These specific runs can be applied to racing distances from 5K to marathon and are done on hard training days. When scheduling workouts, remember you want to alternate easy and hard days—always avoid two hard days in a row.

Pushing Your
Anaerobic Threshold

The Consistent Winning anaerobic threshold run involves running at the fastest pace you can while still maintaining your breathing relatively comfortably. This point is also what is known as the ventilation breaking point—the point where the oxygen supply to your muscles is insufficient for the demands you're placing on them. Anaerobic threshold training helps to elevate the exercise intensity at which you reach oxygen debt. It is one of the best methods for increasing heart efficiency.

The specific purpose of the anaerobic threshold workout is to develop endurance and raise your aerobic capacity. This workout develops your stride, strength, leg speed, and metabolic waste disposal as well as your heart. It will do wonders to help you hold a faster pace over the length of a race.

The anaerobic threshold run consists of a 13- to 21-minute hard run, at the brink of creating an oxygen debt most of the way. Before you begin, run a 13-minute, slow warm-up, stretch, and then jog at least 5 more minutes. After this thorough warm-up, you're ready to begin the anaerobic threshold run.

Run for 13 minutes at the fastest pace you can hold while still breathing smoothly. You may need to build up to this time over a few weeks, and you can use fartlek running to help build up. Fartlek is speed play, running at a fast pace for an arbitrary distance or time, then slowing down—alternating speed with a slow pace. You pick an object in the distance and hold a fast pace until you reach it, or run for 30 seconds or a minute or more holding a fast pace.

Gradually work up to 21 minutes of running, but don't run longer at this fast pace. Twenty-one minutes is enough to give a good training effect yet allow recovery for another hard workout two days later. Any longer will only wear you down and cause low-quality workouts for the next few days.

Alternatives to this particular workout include running 5K races on weekends or running three or four 1-mile repeats (after a thorough warm-up). Running these 1-milers is also a good way to project the pace at which you can run a marathon. (See ''Your Marathon Pace'' on page 94).

What This Workout Accomplishes

Proper anaerobic threshold training helps raise the point at which lactic acid significantly increases in the blood. If you run

YOUR MARATHON PACE

To calculate your marathon pace, thoroughly warm up and then run three separate 1-mile runs as strongly as you can. After each run take a 5-minute cool-down and recovery. Figure the average time of the three runs and add 1 minute. This is your projected marathon pace per mile for your current level of training.

For example, if you averaged 7 minutes per mile, then you can plan on sustaining an average of 8 minutes per mile in a marathon, as long as the rest of your training has been adequate. Run these 1-mile repeats once a month so you'll always be familiar with what your marathon pace is at your current level of training.

slowly enough to get all the oxygen your body needs, then the fat and carbohydrates your muscles are using for energy are broken down into carbon dioxide and water. If you exercise hard enough to create an oxygen debt—when your body isn't getting the oxygen it needs—the carbohydrates are broken down into lactic acid, which builds up in the muscles. You want to avoid high levels of lactic acid, which some researchers have linked to fatigue and pain.

By using anaerobic threshold training, you can raise your anaerobic threshold so that you can exercise longer and harder *before* oxygen debt and significant lactic acid buildup occur.

Anaerobic threshold training is also one of the best methods for increasing heart efficiency. It helps increase the amount of blood pumped with each beat, aiding transportation of oxygen to the working muscles. Some researchers have suggested that a well-trained heart can use small amounts of lactic acid for energy during exercise and still maintain pumping efficiency.

Developing Sprinting Power

Sprinting is a specific workout to increase your strength and speed. It also develops power to accelerate, improves your stride, and helps with metabolic waste disposal. Your muscles increase their ability to keep working under the adverse biochemical conditions created during the physical stress of racing.

Sprinting is also highly specific training aimed at getting your legs moving above and beyond the call of duty. If you practice running a series of 100-yard sprints in 15 seconds, for example, your legs learn to move at a 4:20-per-mile pace. This training effect also carries over to help make your anaerobic threshold runs or 5K races faster and easier. Sprints in combination with anaerobic threshold runs help decrease your marathon time.

Speedwork of any kind, however, must be approached carefully and gradually so you don't get injured. You should train with fartlek running before attempting sprints. By doing this, you build up a tolerance to speedwork gradually without overdoing it.

These three steps will make your sprint workouts safer and more beneficial.

1. Build a base of at least 21 miles a week over a seven- to eight-month period.
2. Add fartlek or speed play to your regular running.
3. Wait until five weeks before your event to begin sprints.

High-Quality Sprint Workouts

Before a sprint workout, you must take time to warm up. This is an absolute requirement before sprint training to help avoid injury. Do the full warm-up outlined in chapter 12, including stretches. Then run another 13 to 21 minutes, including some fartlek-type running. This all adds up to at least 40 minutes of preparation so your body core temperature will increase and your muscles will be thoroughly warmed up.

For your sprint workout, start with a series of three to five 110-yard sprints and progress over a five-week period to eight or ten 110s, depending on your conditioning and ability. Some elite runners go through 12 to 16 220-yard sprints in training for races. It takes the average human about 5 or 6 seconds to reach maximum speed, so don't bother blasting off when you start—this only increases your chances of getting hurt. Run the first two sprints relatively easily.

If you're sprinting with friends, wait until the third sprint to try competing with them. You don't need to run any of the sprints as if your life depended on it, but give it a good effort. Concentrate on form, and try to flow and be smooth. Take 1 or 2 minutes for recovery after each one. You can catch your breath while jogging and walking back to the starting line. Avoid standing around; keep moving to avoid the harmful effects of cooling down too quickly.

Sprints can be fun, especially when done with friends. Make sure that you're well trained but not overtrained when you begin, and you'll look forward to your sprint sessions.

If you are a competition sprinter, the double 3-Month Cycle is ideal for building up explosive strength for sprint competition. Hill work can add more power.

Running to Carbohydrate Depletion

The carbohydrate depletion run is specific for increasing endurance. This is an aerobic run—meaning that it uses oxygen to burn body fuel and provide energy—and it helps endurance by improving oxygen uptake and training your body to burn fat. This helps get you past the approximately 2-hour burnout time in a long event, when the glycogen supplying your muscles with fuel becomes depleted. When someone "hits the wall" or burns out during a long run or race, it frequently happens near this 2-hour point (although it ranges from 1½ to 2½ hours). What happens is that the muscle stores of glycogen become depleted and the fuel supply available for muscle work drops. After this, glycogen from the liver is the major source of glucose, which supplies energy.

You can minimize or eliminate this "wall" by increasing

your workouts to a run of 2 hours plus 15 to 30 minutes at a relatively slow pace each week. The extra 15 to 30 minutes on those slow training runs gets your body used to running beyond 2 hours and develops efficient muscle and liver glycogen stores and metabolism.

It isn't necessary to train at a very fast pace for long runs. Lyn Brooks, who proved herself one of the better female runners in triathlons and ultra-marathons, never trains more than 18 miles, and at a moderate pace. She won the three-day Ultraman Triathlon in 1984 by running the final 53-mile segment nonstop using this type of training and the Consistent Winning timing technique.

The carbohydrate depletion run is long, slow distance. The pace should be 2 to 3 minutes slower than your projected marathon race pace. John Treacy, who won the silver medal in the 1984 Olympic marathon with a fabulous time of 2:09:56, trained at an 8-minute pace for 20 miles on his weekly long run, yet averaged less than 5 minutes per mile in the race!

Carbohydrate depletion workouts in any sport also help weight loss. Your body learns to burn fat more efficiently while doing submaximal aerobic training. You burn calories very efficiently during aerobic training. This is because oxygen is used efficiently to burn fat and carbohydrate in the mitochondria, the powerhouses in our muscle cells, which increase threefold in size and number with aerobic training. An alternative to running for carbohydrate depletion is to occasionally go for a long, easy bicycle ride, which you should also build up to gradually.

During a long run is _not_ the time to push hard. Pushing too hard at the wrong time burns you out unnecessarily. It decreases your ability to do quality workouts over the next few days and thus decreases the overall training effect. You'll lose in the "long run" if you push too hard too often.

Selecting Your Workout

These specific training runs all help to increase aerobic capacity, endurance, and average running speed, three things that surely will benefit your running performance.

When choosing your workouts, individual differences in training, conditioning, and ability must be considered. Some people can recover from a hard day more quickly than others; some people are more naturally adapted to endurance, others to speed. You could choose one or two of the specific runs and vary or combine them.

If your race distance is 5K or 10K, lower the mileage of the anaerobic threshold run and add more intensity by increasing the frequency of your sprints and your anaerobic threshold runs toward race day. You may want to average 1½ to 2 sprint workouts or anaerobic threshold runs a week instead of putting in long miles. If you use those specific runs to enhance your performance, remember to use the easy/hard principle when outlining schedules.

Novice runners should begin specific training by building base mileage and working gradually into fartlek runs before incorporating the anaerobic threshold or sprint workouts.

For someone beginning specific training, the anaerobic threshold run is the first choice for improvement in any shorter distance race, and the carbohydrate depletion run is the first choice for a marathon. Sprints are the last choice for relative newcomers to racing.

CHAPTER FIFTEEN

MENTAL TECHNIQUES

Throughout the recorded history of mankind, no runner broke the 4-minute mile until 1954. After Roger Bannister broke the historic barrier, 50 other runners also did so in the next year and a half. To a large extent, that barrier had been only in the mind.

Once other runners knew that Bannister could do a sub-4-minute mile, they began to think that they could, too. They could "see" themselves doing it. The solution was a mental one.

This chapter is designed to help you with mental strategy and psychological techniques so you can optimize your performances. You already know how powerful the mind can be in its influence over the body. Anxiety, worry, and negative thinking certainly have degenerative effects on the body and will impair your performance. Psychological stress has physiological consequences. Arteries constrict, blood pressure elevates, and muscles may cramp from the decreased blood flow. An athlete dwelling on his or her last mistake may "choke" because the worrying has now caused physical handicaps. Longer-term by-products of negative thinking include upset stomach, headaches, ulcers, shingles, and so on.

If you have positive thoughts or think about the things you really want, however, the effects are then positive. You feel more relaxed, the body helps heal itself, and you perform better. Studies of high achievers in sports show consistently that they virtually "eat, sleep, and breathe" their goals. There is no room to crowd in a negative thought. They have seen their goals over and over in their mind so many times that, during competition, they can focus on the action intensely enough that the rest of the world ceases to exist. Their performance seems to happen automatically.

Many of us are great at worrying—what we need to do is make an effort to put in more mental time on the positive side. It has long been said that whether you think you *can* or think you *can't*—you're right.

Visualization—A Goal in Sight

Good visualization technique involves seeing in your mind what you want. If you want positive results, you need to start seeing things in that light. You can expand the visualizing part of your mind by using it more vividly. See, hear, feel, smell, taste, and live your victory or goal in your mind in every detail you can imagine. Rehearse in your mind how you want things to be. Imagination is somewhat different than visualization: Imagination is the first time you see something in your mind, and visualization is recalling something you have already imagined or have seen in real life.

Goal setting makes your expectations more clear. It also increases your motivation, self-confidence, and focus. To attain a goal, you must give something to attain it. It helps to see in your mind's eye what you're willing to give. This additional detail helps further create the path of action you have already begun.

Maxwell Maltz said in his book *Psycho-Cybernetics,* "You act and feel, not according to what things are really like, but according to the image your mind holds of what they are like." The brain decodes nerve impulses that our senses pick up from the environment, and we perceive them as ideas or mental images that we react to or interact with.

If you are casually riding a bicycle, for example, and suddenly a dog charges at you, your senses have provided you with a mental image that causes you to react. Adrenaline is pumped into your bloodstream, giving you new power to get away. You react and function from what your mind perceives, whether it's real or not. For instance, if you only dreamed this incident, you might awaken with pounding heart.

Mental rehearsal allows you to practice new endeavors, such as athletic performances. How you perceive yourself, whether in a positive or negative way, affects your reactions. Golf instructor Alex Morrison used to say, ''You must have a clear mental picture of the correct thing before you can do it successfully.''

Visualization helps guide your physiology in a constructive direction during training and competition. With it you can learn to relax and overcome worrying your way to indigestion and other negative physiological effects that may cause you to ''choke'' during an event.

How Does It Work?

Vivid imagination and visualization take place at lower brain wave frequencies—or alpha waves—that we produce when relaxing, sleeping, or meditating. Research has shown that at the lower brain wave frequencies, the mind is in a very receptive state. This receptive, subjective part of the mind usually does not distinguish between what is real and what is vividly imagined. Have you ever had a very realistic dream that seemed utterly ridiculous once you awakened and thought about it in your conscious, objective mind? The subjective, and sometimes subconscious, part of the mind is a storehouse for information and makes no judgments about any of it. That's up to the objective part of the mind.

What exactly are these brain waves? Scientists measure the electrical activity of the brain with an electroencephalograph, or EEG. The activity ranges in frequency from less than 1 cycle per second to about 21 cycles per second (CPS) and is divided into several levels. From about 14 to 21 CPS, in the higher (beta) waves, the mind is mostly in an objective broadcast mode. You do most of your talking when your mind is in this cycle. In alpha, about 7 to 14 CPS, which is the middle of the brain wave spectrum, the mind is primarily in a subjective receptive mode. The middle of alpha, 10½ CPS, is the center of the whole spectrum, and for thousands of years man has experienced this type of brain wave as a special relaxed state—meditation.

When the brain is in the alpha range, the mind may be aware of its surroundings but can still be daydreaming and in a very relaxed state. Most of the time spent in the alpha range, people are asleep and dreaming. This is also known as the rapid eye movement (REM) phase of sleep. Most of us also have experienced the alpha range while in deep daydreams. Have you ever been driving on the highway when suddenly you "wake up" to realize that you've traveled past several exits you didn't notice? Your mind was in the alpha range, but you weren't actually asleep.

With a little practice you can train yourself to expand this consciousness or conscious functioning by remaining awake in alpha and deriving the benefits this state of mind offers. Visualizing something while your brain is in the alpha state is many times more effective than thinking of it when you're fully awake.

At the faster beta brain waves, it appears that the mind broadcasts, or puts into physical use, what was put into it at the lower brain waves. Therefore, you can take advantage of what you "programmed" at the lower alpha waves. This phenomenon was used by East German athletes at the last several Olympics, as noted by Charles Garfield in his book *Peak Performance,* and is used by many elite athletes today. Creatively visualizing your desired end result, particularly at relaxed states, can program you into physically creating your previous mental picture. You are now, to a certain degree, in charge of your own physiology.

How to Do It

This is a fundamental exercise that will train your mind and body to be responsive to your own mental images, which is most efficiently done with your brain in the alpha state. There are many schools of thought on how to relax. Most are practically adapted to the individual's belief system. Basically what is required is finding a comfortable place (preferably not lying down), breathing correctly, and practicing a simple countdown exercise. Don't be concerned if you fall sleep the first few times; you'll get better at it. These are the most important steps for preparing your mind for the relaxation mode.

Correct breathing for relaxation is diaphragmatic or belly breathing. Breathe deeply in through your nose and extend the lower abdomen, which helps you pull the diaphragm down. The lower part of the lungs fill with air. Then expand the chest, filling the upper part of the lungs. Let the air out slowly. You've probably noticed how deep sighs help you relax. Controlled breathing also helps mental focus.

Start at 100, 50, or 25, and mentally count backward, visualizing and hearing each number in your mind. A method that works well for many people is to imagine walking down a staircase, with each step numbered in descending order. Then imagine achieving your desired goals, whether it's lifting a certain weight or running a certain time in a race. Actually *see* yourself doing everything you desire in vivid details, both through your own eyes and as if you're watching yourself as a spectator. It is important to see what you want. It's best to keep visualization in a realm that you, in your objective beta mind, believe may be possible.

What you are doing is projecting into the future by creating it in the present. For example, the book you are holding in your hand was an imagined idea (projected into the future) before it came into existence. The same is true for the clothes on your body and the chair or sofa you are sitting on right now. They were all imagined before they were created. Use imagination and visualization to create positive goals. The subconscious mind stores whatever images, thoughts, and goals you put into it, and subconsciously it leads you in that direction.

Imagination and visualization give you definite direction, a destiny. Take the time to set a destination or goal so the right side of your brain can help you. It is said that a ship without a destination has no favoring winds. No matter which way the wind blows, it is of no help if the ship isn't being steered. When you know where you're going, the means to get there will fall into place. At first, visualizing goals may seem difficult or your images silly, but if you don't clearly see your goals it will be difficult if not impossible to ever reach them. How can things go your way if you don't know where you're going?

Putting It into Practice

You can practice by visualizing anything in detail, such as an apple. Visualize an apple and vividly describe it. It's a deep red McIntosh with some tinges of yellow interspersed over the surface, and it has a smooth, shiny texture. The lower half is slightly narrower in circumference than the upper half. As its shape curves inward at the top and bottom, it becomes involuted. A brown stem, somewhat thickened on the end, comes out of the top involution. There are two bright green leaves coming off the stem, both with serrated edges and pointed at the end. Its juicy, pale yellow interior has a delicious, mouth-watering sweetness that makes your salivary glands tingle.

Getting the idea? You have to see it to say it. The more details, the better. Mental conditioning is an exercise like your workouts. You get better with practice.

Now see yourself training and getting stronger. Picture yourself at the race. You're warmed up, stretched out, ready. Your muscles are moving smoothly and efficiently. You're determined, relaxed, fast, competing at your planned pace, doing your own race. Feel your muscles, leg movement, arm movement, breathing. You're passing other competitors right and left, executing planned strategy, setting a personal record, winning. Hear the sounds, feel the wind, taste the sweat trickling down your face, smell the air...

We see you doing it, too.

CHAPTER SIXTEEN

ANSWERING YOUR QUESTIONS

Wondering just how Consistent Winning will fit into your sports schedule? Here are answers to questions that athletes frequently ask.

Q. What if I only train three days a week—can I still use Consistent Winning?

A. Yes. To peak for an event, begin with the 3-Week Cycle, working out three days a week until the last week. Then alter your training to set up a 3-Day Cycle. During the training days of the 3-Day Cycle, train moderately the first day, easy the second day, and go all out the third day (your competition day). If you are on a strict three-day-a-week workout schedule, only working out every other day, make your third workout of the week (after two consecutive days off) the hard one.

When beginning the workouts for the 3-Week Cycle, try to work out the first few days in a row to get your body and the cycles going. Then settle in to three days a week, the third workout of the week being the hard one.

Q. What cycle should I use if my next event is only two weeks away?

A. The 3-Day Cycle. Assuming that you already have a good training base, continue training until five days before the event. Use the 3-Day Cycle's taper-down, starting five days before the event. Take two rest days, and then taper up on the last two days directly before the event. You will peak on the next day, the day of your event.

Q. What if I only have seven weeks or nine weeks until my event? How do I schedule it?

A. Count back on a calendar as though you were using a 3-Month Cycle. If there are nine weeks before your event, count back from the event day and mark in the 3-Day and 3-Week Cycles. Continue counting back another five weeks for training and three days for resting, and begin your cycle there. If you only have seven weeks before your event, use two 3-Week Cycles in a row and include the 3-Day Cycle at the end.

Q. What if I have repeated clusters of competitions, such as two three-day events, two or three days apart?

A. When you have competition three days in a row followed by two or three days' rest and then three days of competition again, you can extend your peak performance to cover the multiple-day competitions. Set up a 3-Week and 3-Day Cycle to peak the first day of the first event. After the first three-day event, take a rest day if you've been in strenuous competition. Then taper back up the one or two days to the second three-day event.

Q. If my main sport is running, can I swim laps on a rest day?

A. You can't swim laps on a rest day if you want a training period to end with a peak performance. The constant activity of lap swimming has an aerobic training effect. The Consistent Winning definition of rest means no aerobic or anaerobic exercise. The rest days are important because they are timed to "set up" a training peak. If you have to do something on a rest day, take a 20- to 30-minute walk. If you must, some nonaerobic, easy-going recreational exercise is okay.

Q. Will these cycles work for anything other than sports?

A. Yes, these cycles are modeled after patterns found throughout nature and will work for any type of performance, such as singing, playing music, dancing, creating art, military training, and industrial applications. They will even work for racehorses: Frequently racehorses will run faster times in qualifications than they will in the race. The horses are peaking too soon.

Q. Is it okay to use a five-day resting period between two 3-Month Cycles instead of 13 days?

A. To set up the 3-Month Cycle, it's important to detrain for the 13 days for maximum effect. In a pinch, you may try only a five-day rest, but the effect will not be as great on your next peak.

Q. If there isn't enough time to do a complete 3-Month Cycle, can I cut out some of the resting days?

A. Cutting out some of the resting days is counterproductive because your catapult effect will not be as great as if you detrained properly. As long as you have a training base, you're better off cutting out training days. If you have to cut out resting days, be sure that two rest days precede your training period.

Q. What if I want to keep track of my own cycles *before* I decide to change my training schedule. What should I record?

A. Use a calendar to record your training days. Record when you train and when you rest. Rate each day subjectively, using a scale of 1 to 5, with ''3'' being an average good day and ''5'' being a great day. Also record the distance, time, or relative intensity of your workout. Many people also like to keep track of their resting pulse rate, usually before getting up in the morning.

Q. Wouldn't it be better to train than stress out during an extended rest?

A. No! A resting period is not a ''stress out'' because there are never more than two complete rest days in a row. In extended resting periods, there are active rest days between rest days.

Q. How intense should training be during a taper-up period?

A. Easy the first day back and easy to moderate the second day back, depending on how much endurance is required on the third or event day. The third day will be a peak day. Intensity is also relative to your individual ability and what you consider your maximum performance.

Q. Suppose I'm in a tournament and have a day off between events?

A. Use a complete 3-Day Cycle leading up to the first event day. Then, depending on how many days of competition you have before the day off, continue with very easy to moderate training on the day between events.

Q. Does someone using Consistent Winning have good performances because they are totally psyched up thinking they have an edge—but they're actually benefiting only from positive thinking?

A. Most athletes can recall entering a competition with high enthusiasm, being totally psyched up and doing well. They can also recall entering competition totally psyched up and doing poorly. As mentioned before, peak performances frequently come a few days too early or a few days too late, if at all, if you're not using timed cycles of resting and training. The Consistent Winning technique helps control physiological and mental response. Consistent Winning allows for and gives you a physical and mental rest to make sure you are ready for a peak performance. Mental techniques and mental state do definitely *help* produce superior performances and are addressed in chapter 15.

GLOSSARY

aerobic metabolism. Use of oxygen to burn body fuel, mostly fat and carbohydrate, and provide energy for exercise.

Aikido. A martial art harmonizing energy in natural circular or spiral patterns.

anaerobic. During exercise, production of energy without using oxygen; limited to short periods of time.

anaerobic threshold. (also lactate turning point and ventilation breaking point) Used here as a point near which the oxygen supply to the muscles is insufficient for their demands; the maximum exercise effort sustainable without getting "out of breath."

atrophy. Wasting away or decrease in size of tissue.

burnout. Mental staleness, loss of vigor, and a feeling of fatigue that result from overtraining without adequate resting periods.

catapult effect. A rebound to a peak performance from resting or detraining after an adequate training base has been built.

Chaos theory. Explanation of patterns evident in behavior or natural occurrences that were previously thought to be irregular and erratic.

Consistent Winning. An adjunct to training that uses timing cycles in harmony with nature to produce continuing success while helping to avoid injury, illness, and burnout.

Consistent Winning technique. The application of natural mathematical patterns to maximize performance.

Cycles. *3-Day Cycle*—A resting period of three days or more (taper-down) followed by three days of training (taper-up), with maximum performance on the third day. *3-Week Cycle*—A resting period of five days or more followed by 21 days of training with maximum performance on the 21st day. (The 3-Day Cycle overlaps the final six days.) *3-Month Cycle*—A resting period of 13 days or more followed by 12 weeks of training with maximum performance on the 84th day.

cytochrome c. An enzyme, or chemical substance, in muscle cells that helps generate energy for aerobic metabolism.

divine proportion. *See* golden mean

Elliott Wave Principle. Graphic interpretation of natural cyclic patterns of social or crowd behavior based on Fibonacci numbers; first described by R. N. Elliott in 1934.

exercise physiology. The study of the changes in the function of the body during and after physical exertion.

exercise psychobiology. The study of the changes in mind/body interaction during and after physical exertion.

fartlek. Speed play, a burst of speed for a variable distance during a training run.

Fibonacci numbers. A natural progression of numbers created by making each number the sum of the two preceding numbers; 1, 1, 2, 3, 5, 8, 13, 21, 34, 55, 89, 144, 233, 377...

fractal geometry. A mathematical language describing families of shapes in which each level or progression shows a similar or identical pattern, but in a different scale.

glycerol. The structure to which fatty acids are attached to form triglycerides. Glycerol is present in chemical combination in most stored body fats.

glycogen. Substance formed that stores carbohydrates in the muscle and liver cells for future conversion to sugar that can be used for muscle activity or generating heat.

golden mean. The point that divides a shape or form into two parts that have a ratio of 0.618:1 to each other.

golden proportion. (also golden ratio) The ratio of one Fibonacci number to either the one preceeding or following it, which equals either 0.618:1 or 1.618:1.

golden spiral. An expanding curve, as in a nautilus shell, where the radii of any diameter are in 0.618:1 relationship to each other.

harmonic proportion. A ratio or mathematical function that repeats itself in a pattern, such as the Fibonacci or golden ratio, 0.618:1 or 1.618:1.

lactic acid. (also lactate) A by-product of anaerobic metabolism; formed during muscular activity by the breakdown of glycogen, a type of sugar stored in the liver and in muscle.

maximum oxygen uptake (VO_2 max). The amount of oxygen the body uses at maximum workload; a measure of endurance training or physical fitness.

mitochondria. The powerhouses in the muscle cells where chemicals that contain energy for muscular work are created through aerobic metabolism; this is where oxygen is used to burn fat. Endurance training increases size and number of mitochondria.

overtraining. Too much training, possibly leading to psychological and physiological problems such as irritability, loss of sleep, and possibly mental or physical burnout.

peak performance. The maximum performance obtainable from the amount of training done.

period. A specific length of time for resting or for training.

periodization. An Eastern European training system used in an attempt to maximize performance with two cycles per year.

phi ratio. (also phi function) 0.618 or 1.618:1; phi $= (\sqrt{5} +$ or $-1) \div 2$. This equals 1.618 and 0.618. *See also* golden mean

podiatry. The specialized medical and surgical practice of restoring healthy function to the lower extremities.

rest base. Sufficient recovery time in a trained individual to allow a rebound to a peak performance or "catapult effect."

resting. *Active rest*—About 20 to 30 minutes of easy training on a day during a resting period. *Rest*—Resting completely or doing another low-intensity activity (such as walking) for 20 to 30 minutes. No training and no practicing your particular activity.

sports psychology. The study of personality and changes in mood of athletes during and after physical exertion.

stress. Any challenge, physical or psychological, to balanced body function or homeostasis.

taper-down. A period of decreased training leading to a rest; the resting period of the 3-Day Cycle.

taper-up. A three-day period of increased training after a resting period; the last three days and training period of the 3-Day Cycle.

timing cycle. A balanced combination of resting and training.

tolerance to exercise. A decreased sensitivity to repeated exercise, sometimes creating a need to increase the amount of training in order to satisfy the same psychological craving; this may not allow for recovery and may lead to injury, illness, and burnout.

training. Practice and conditioning to develop abilities of the body and mind. Easy, moderate, and hard training degrees vary with time and intensity and are subject to interpretation based on individual experience.

training base. The foundation of physical conditioning established over time, from which a peak performance can be generated.

triglyceride. A common fat found in food and stored in the body; it consists of three fatty acids attached to a glycerol core. Triglycerides, produced in the liver from carbohydrates, make up a large portion of the fatty substances in the blood.

VO$_2$ max. *See* maximum oxygen uptake

warm-up. The increase of body temperature, circulation, and flexibility by slow exercise including stretching.

RESOURCES

Math, Fibonacci Numbers, and the Elliott Wave

Barnsley, Michael. *Fractals Everywhere*. Boston: Academic Press, 1988.

Bohm, David, and F. David Peat. *Science, Order, Creativity*. Toronto: Bantam, 1987.

Brenneman, Richard J., ed. *Fuller's Earth: A Day with Bucky and the Kids*. New York: St. Martin's Press, 1984.

Cook, Theodore A. *The Curves of Life*. New York: Dover, 1979.

Doczi, Gyorgy. *The Power of Limits*. Boston: Shambhala, 1981.

Ghyka, Matila. *The Geometry of Art and Life*. New York: Dover, 1978.

Gleick, James. *Chaos: Making a New Science*. New York: Penguin Books, 1988.

Grunbaum, Branko, and G. C. Shephard. *Tilings and Patterns*. New York: W. H. Freeman, 1986.

Hambidge, Jay. *Elements of Dynamic Symmetry.* New York: Dover, 1967.

Hofstadter, Douglas R. *Godel, Escher, Bach: An Eternal Golden Braid.* New York: Basic Books, 1979.

Huntley, H. E. *Divine Proportion: A Study in Mathematical Beauty.* New York: Dover, 1970.

Lawlor, Robert. *Sacred Geometry: Philosophy and Practice.* New York: Thames & Hudson, 1989.

Luce, Gay Gaer. *Body Time: Physiological Rhythms and Social Stress.* New York: Pantheon Books, 1971.

Mandelbrot, Benoit B. *The Fractal Geometry of Nature.* New York: W. H. Freeman, 1982.

Polkinghorne, John. *Science and Creation.* Boston: Shambhala, 1989.

Prechter, Robert R., Jr., and R. N. Elliott. *The Major Works of R. N. Elliott.* Chappaqua, N.Y.: New Classics, 1984.

Prechter, Robert R., Jr., and Alfred J. Frost. *Elliott Wave Principle: Key to Stock Market Profits.* Chappaqua, N.Y.: New Classics, 1985.

Purce, Jill. *The Mystic Spiral: Journey of the Soul.* New York: Thames & Hudson, 1987.

Rucker, Rudolf V. *Geometry, Relativity, and the Fourth Dimension.* New York: Dover, 1977.

Rucker, Rudy. *Mind Tools: The Five Levels of Mathematical Reality.* Boston: Houghton Mifflin, 1988.

Winfree, Arthur T. *The Timing of Biological Clocks.* New York: W. H. Freeman, 1987.

Zee, Anthony. *Fearful Symmetry: The Search for Beauty in Modern Physics.* New York: Macmillan, 1986.

Sports Performance

Artal, Raul, and Robert A. Wiswell. *Exercise in Pregnancy.* Baltimore: Williams & Wilkins, 1985.

Bompa, Tudor O. *Theory and Methodology of Training: The Key to Athletic Performance.* Dubuque, Iowa: Kendall/Hunt, 1983.

Edwards, Sally. *Triathlon: A Triple Fitness Sport.* Chicago: Contemporary Books, 1983.

Glover, Bob, and Pete Schuder. *The New Competitive Runner's Handbook.* New York: Penguin Books, 1988.

Konopka, Peter. *The Complete Cycle Sport Guide.* Wakefield, England: EP Publishing Ltd., 1982.

Marino, John, Lawrence May, and Hal Z. Bennett. *John Marino's Bicycling Book.* Los Angeles: J. P. Tarcher, 1981.

Mirkin, Gabe, and Marshall Hoffman. *The Sportsmedicine Book.* Boston: Little, Brown, 1978.

Nieman, David C. *Fitness and Sports Medicine: An Introduction.* Palo Alto, Calif.: Bull Publishing, 1990.

Noakes, Tim. *Lore of Running.* Champaign, Ill.: Leisure Press, 1991.

Stegemann, Jurgen. *Exercise Physiology.* Chicago: Medical Year Book, 1981.

Subotnick, Steven, ed. *Sports Medicine of the Lower Extremity.* New York: Churchill Livingstone, 1988.

Van Aaken, Ernst. *The Van Aaken Method.* Mountain View, Calif.: Anderson World, 1976.

Wells, Christine L. *Women, Sport, and Performance.* Champaign, Ill.: Human Kinetics, 1985.

Wilmore, Jack H., and David L. Costill. *Training for Sport and Activity: The Physiological Basis of the Conditioning Process.* Dubuque, Iowa: William C. Brown, 1988.

Mental Techniques

Benson, Herbert, and Miriam Z. Klipper. _The Relaxation Response_. New York: Avon, 1976.

Garfield, Charles A., and Hal Z. Bennett. _Peak Performance: Mental Training Techniques of the World's Greatest Athletes_. Los Angeles: J. P. Tarcher, 1984.

Harris, Dorothy V., and Bette L. Harris. _The Athlete's Guide to Sports Psychology: Mental Skills for Physical People_. New York: Leisure Press, 1984.

Hudson, Thomas J. _The Law of Psychic Phenomena_. San Jose, Calif.: Institute for Human Growth, 1970.

Maltz, Maxwell. _Psycho-Cybernetics_. New York: Pocket Books, 1983.

Murphy, Michael, and Rhea A. White. _The Psychic Side of Sports_. Reading, Mass.: Addison-Wesley, 1978.

Selye, Hans. _The Stress of Life_. New York: McGraw-Hill, 1956.

Silva, John M. III, and Robert S. Weinberg, eds. _Psychological Foundations of Sport_. Champaign, Ill.: Human Kinetics, 1984.

Silva, José. _The Silva Mind Control Method_. New York: Pocket Books, 1978.

Suinn, Richard M. _Psychology in Sports: Methods and Applications_. Minneapolis: Burgess, 1980.

Suinn, Richard M. _Seven Steps to Peak Performance_. Toronto: Hans Huber, 1987.

Syer, John, and Christopher Connolly. _Sporting Body, Sporting Mind: An Athlete's Guide to Mental Training_. Englewood Cliffs, N.J.: Prentice Hall, 1988.

Tutko, Thomas A., and Umberto Tosi. _Sports Psyching: Playing Your Best Game All of the Time_. Los Angeles: J. P. Tarcher, 1976.

ABOUT
THE AUTHORS

Ronald D. Sandler, D.P.M.

Ronald D. Sandler, D.P.M., who discovered and developed the Consistent Winning technique, is a practitioner of podiatric medicine and surgery and training consultant based in Houston, Texas. He earned his degree at the Ohio College of Podiatric Medicine in Cleveland. He practiced podiatry in Cheyenne, Wyoming, where he was appointed vice chairman of the Board of Registration in Podiatry by the governor. It was there that he developed the mathematical model for Consistent Winning in 1982.

Because he is an athlete himself, Dr. Sandler has been sought out by many injured athletes seeking a sports medicine specialist. He has lectured to many clubs and groups on the subjects of running, walking, bicycling, general fitness, and competitive sports. Dr. Sandler has traveled extensively to athletic events, including the Ironman Triathlon in Hawaii, to do research and to help athletes using Consistent Winning. He is a member of the American College of Sports Medicine and the American Academy of Podiatric Sports Medicine. He works out regularly doing weight

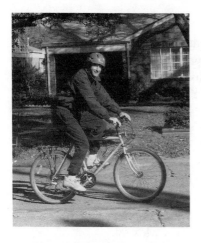

Dr. Ronald Sandler regularly uses Consistent Winning to prepare for bicycle centuries.

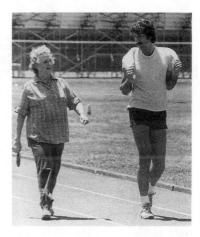

Dr. Dennis Lobstein, here with one of his adult fitness program participants, has created exercise programs for many groups.

training, using StairMaster, hiking, and training for annual 100-mile bicycle rides.

Dennis D. Lobstein, Ph.D.

Dennis D. Lobstein, Ph.D., is an exercise psychobiologist, physiologist, and private consultant based near Albuquerque, New Mexico. His doctoral training was under the direction of A. H. Ismail, H.S.D. (doctor of health science), at Purdue University. He also studied athletic training and sports medicine at Northwestern University Medical School's Center for Sports Medicine.

Dr. Lobstein is a former professor of exercise physiology at the University of New Mexico in Albuquerque, where he was director of the Exercise Biochemistry Laboratory and the Adult Fitness Program. His areas of expertise include adult fitness, human performance, and exercise psychobiology. He has done fitness testing and created exercise programs for many institutions and groups, including the New Mexico Law Enforcement Academy, paramedics, and government personnel. Dr. Lobstein has presented research in Austria, Japan, China, and throughout the United States. His research, published in numerous journals, includes physical fitness and the biochemistry of emotional stability, exercise addiction, and martial arts fitness systems. Dr. Lobstein has been involved with martial arts and the study of mind/body interaction for more than 20 years.

Dr. Lobstein is a Fellow of the American College of Sports Medicine and a member of the American Association for the Advancement of Science and Sigma Xi, among other societies. He is a runner who uses Consistent Winning, and he enjoys frequent hikes in the mountains of New Mexico.

INDEX

Note: Page references in *italic* indicate illustrations.